Going Blind

Going Blind

A Memoir

MARA FAULKNER, OSB

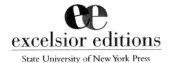

excelsior editions
State University of New York Press
Albany, New York

Cover photo courtesy of the author (private collection).

Published by
State University of New York Press, Albany

© 2009 State University of New York

Excelsior Editions is an imprint of State University of New York Press

For information, contact State University of New York Press, Albany, NY
www.sunypress.edu

Production by Eileen Meehan
Marketing by Anne M. Valentine

Library of Congress Cataloging-in-Publication Data

Faulkner, Mara.
    Going blind : a memoir / Mara Faulkner.
        p. cm.
    Includes bibliographical references and index.
    ISBN 978-1-4384-2667-9 (hardcover : alk. paper)
    ISBN 978-1-4384-2668-6 (pbk. : alk. paper)
    1. Faulkner, Mara.   2. Children of blind parents—United States—Biography.
I. Title.

    HQ759.912.F38 2009
    306.874'2092—dc22

    [B]   2008046865

10 9 8 7 6 5 4 3 2 1

I dedicate Going Blind *to my father and mother,*
Dennis Faulkner and Hattie Miller Faulkner.
Though they died many years ago, their lives teach me
daily lessons about endurance, laughter, a beautiful frugality,
and the courage to question. They are the heart of this book,
and my greatest hope is that I did justice in writing about them.

Contents

Acknowledgments

I thank my brother and sisters—Dennis Faulkner, Judy Faulkner McGuire, Jeanne Adelmeyer, Elaine Willenbring, Coreen Faulkner, and Mona Faulkner. Any of them could have written a version of this book, but instead they entrusted their memories and experiences to me. My nephews Jeb Willenbring and Chad McGuire patiently answered my many questions. All of them, plus other nieces and nephews, read drafts and offered helpful suggestions. I also thank my rigorous, generous readers who stuck with me through the ten long years this book has taken: Karen Erickson, Anne Patrick, SNJM, Nancy Hynes, OSB, Julie Kellum Jensen, Patrick Henry, Monza Naff, and Judy McGuire, my first, last, and best editor. Travel and research were possible because of a Central Minnesota Arts Board grant and travel grants from the College of St. Benedict. I am grateful for the hospitable space at Hedgebrook and Soapstone writers' retreats and the St. Benedict's Monastery Studium. Laura Schwarz, my faithful, cheerful researcher and typist, has hunted up numerous citations and typed endless drafts and revisions. At SUNY Press, I'd like to thank Larin McLaughlin, Eileen Meehan, Andrew Kenyon, and Susan Petrie for enthusiasm and reliable, skillful help.

ACKNOWLEDGMENTS

My Benedictine community, and especially the women I live with, have influenced me in more ways than I can name. Most important, their values have helped me see my parents, my family, and even blindness more clearly and lovingly.

This book belongs to these people and many others. To all of you, blessings and thanks.

I gratefully acknowledge permission to reprint the following material:

From "My Father's Harmonica." Unpublished poem by Jeanne Adelmeyer. Used by permission of the author.

From "Disability: A Lament." Copyright © 1998 by Helen Betenbaugh and Marjorie Procter-Smith, from "Disabling the Lie: Prayers of Truth and Transformation," in *Human Disability and the Service of God: Reassessing Religious Practice*. Used by permission of Abingdon Press.

From "The Immigrant Irish." Copyright © 1987 by Eavan Boland, from *An Origin like Water: Collected Poems 1967–1987* by Eavan Boland. Used by permission of W. W. Norton & Company, Inc., and Carcanet Press Limited.

From "Christ Be Our Light." Copyright © 1994 Bernadette Farrell, from *Christ Be Our Light* by Bernadette Farrell. Published by OCP Publications, 5536 NE Hassalo, Portland, OR 97213. All rights reserved. Used with permission.

Unpublished haikus by Itaru Ina. Used by permission of Satsuki Ina, PhD.

From *Planet of the Blind* by Stephen Kuusisto, copyright © 1998 by Stephen Kuusisto. Used by permission of the Dial Press/Dell Publishing, a division of Random House, Inc., and Irene Skolnick Literary Agency.

From "Among My Souvenirs" by Edgar Leslie and Horatio Nicholls © 1927 (Renewed) Chappell & Co. Inc., and Edgar Leslie.

ACKNOWLEDGMENTS

All Rights Reserved. Used by permission of Alfred Publishing Co., Inc. and Herald Square Music, Inc. on behalf of Edgar Leslie.

From "World of Our Own." Words and Music by Tom Springfield © 1965 (Renewed) Springfield-Music, Ltd. All Rights Administered by Chappell Music Ltd. All Rights Reserved. Used by permission of Alfred Publishing Co., Inc.

Glory be to you, O God of the night,
for the whiteness of the moon
and the infinite stretches of dark space.
Let me be learning to love the night
as I know and love the day.
Let me be learning to trust the darkness
and to seek its subtle blessings.
Let me be learning the night's way of seeing
that in all things I may trace the mystery
of your presence.

—J. Philip Newell, *Celtic Benediction*

ONE

Blind Spot

The small, circular, optically insensitive region in the retina where fibers of the optic nerve emerge from the eyeball. It has no rods or cones. A subject about which one is markedly ignorant or prejudicial.

BLINDNESS WAS MY father's blind spot, and it became my family's and mine, the word we didn't dare say. In our house there was no gentle, businesslike dog, no white cane, no Braille playing cards or talking books. Rather than accepting and adapting to his blindness, my father, Dennis Faulkner, hoped and prayed for a cure—though less and less as the years went by—and walked a step behind my mother, an unobtrusive hand on her arm. In the early days, he made a game of not being able to see. Because there were seven kids in our family, he often dressed my little sisters. His hands were gentle with them as he held them one by one between his knees and pulled on panties, long stockings, and high white shoes. He couldn't see which shoe fit which foot, but he always made a game of it. "Right-er-left-er-left-er-right?" he'd ask. They'd giggle with delighted superiority and set him straight.

Somewhere along the way, the games and laughter ended, and instead of jokes about blindness, we silently agreed on denial, learning vigilance to help preserve his illusion. We whisked obstacles—the dog, little kids, footstools—out of his way and put cups and tools into his hands, so he wouldn't have to ask or grope. One Sunday when the nine of us were walking from the car up the steps to St. Joseph's Catholic Church, a woman who obviously knew us asked me, "Is your daddy blind?"

Feeling as if she had insulted him or accused him of something obscene, I said indignantly, "No, he just can't see too well." All through grade school, high school, and college, I never told a single soul outside my family that I had a blind father, protecting his secret as closely as if he were a gangster or an excon.

Because I lost my father when I was too young to know him, I can only guess why blindness became our secret. I left home at eighteen, fleeing Mandan, North Dakota, my dead little hometown. The college my five sisters, my brother, and I attended was four hundred miles from home, and I had only enough money to go home at Christmas and in the summer. By then, my dad was aging and growing more and more silent. I loved him, but it never occurred to me to be interested in him as a person beyond the one I knew and the earlier one revealed in the stories I'd heard a few times too often.

Then I joined a Benedictine monastery and left him even further behind. As I look now at the stiff, silly letters I wrote home those early years of my monastic life, I realize that I must have found it impossible to bridge the gap between my simple home and the world of prayer, study, and constant cleaning that comprised my first couple of years in the monastery. Once my mother sent me a bag of carrots from her garden, with the dirt still on them. At home, I always ate them that way, straight from the garden, brushing the dirt off on my jeans. But the other novices were getting huge boxes of Fanny Farmer chocolates from their families. I hid my carrots and eventually threw them away. With my mother, I was lucky that she lived past my years of self-absorption and shame and that I chanced upon Tillie Olsen, Grace Paley, and many other working-class feminist writers who helped me see her and her hard-working life in a new light. By the time she died in 1993, I understood her and admired her for a hundred reasons.

My father had no such chance at redemption. He died when I was twenty-five, and my grief for him was buried beneath the stony silence of the novitiate. Shortly after he died, my mother wrote with rare directness, "I know you lost your favorite person." She was right. But in the years that followed, as my mother flourished in reality and in my estimation, my father diminished to a broken shadow who appeared only once in my dreams—an old, thin man in his faded blue sweater, lying on his side, silent, blind, with his big strong hands helpless and useless between his knees. Have you come, old man, I wondered, to lead me after you, cursing, into the darkness?

In doing research on Tillie Olsen, I learned another lesson: smarts and a flair for language come from somewhere. I came to hate the idea of isolated genius, the *onlys*, the woman writer "imprisoned in uniqueness," as Germaine Greer describes it, and to look for visible or invisible evidence of influence and support for the women writers I was studying. It recently occurred to me to look for such evidence in my own history.

So I began this search almost out of curiosity. My five sisters, my brother, and I all have the ability, seemingly untaught, to feel the rhythm and swing of language, to delight in it, and to catch it on paper. Where did this ability come from? Not from our serviceable but unremarkable schools. Not from my mother. The weekly letters she wrote faithfully to her distant children were stream-of-thought sentences, sprawled on the page without much punctuation and with no literary grace. She wrote as associatively as she talked and almost never sat down to read a book.

After my mother died, I finally felt free to read the letters my father wrote to her toward the end of their long courtship. I expected to find there a wild flair for language and a skill like ours. For wasn't our father a great storyteller, and hadn't he recommended Zane Grey's Western romances, which my sisters and I carried home by the bushelful from the public library and read through the long summer days? What I found in those letters, written in a crabbed hand on cheap little tablet pages, is not graceful. The letters are inarticulate, filled with clichés and commonplaces, misspelled words and odd punctuation, words spelled the way the Irish say them (*lave* for *leave*, for instance), and his distress that he couldn't put into written words what he felt for the little blond sweetheart he was courting. Dennis Faulkner (even his name had several spellings—Dennis, Denis, Den) was not a man of the pen; he had none of the linguistic skill of a James Joyce or a Frank O'Connor, nor even of a Louis L'Amour. I was so disappointed in those letters it took me another six years to learn some of what they have to tell me. I won't plunder them for my own uses; they are too personal, too intimate, the long love song of a forty-two-year-old man who sees his last chance of happiness being squeezed to death by poverty and by the post-Depression economy of the late 1930s in Minnesota and North Dakota.

Those letters didn't solve the mystery of my literary heritage, but they showed me another connection between my father and me and brought to light the deeper mystery of his blindness. I was two years old when my father wrote his only letter to me. My mother, my older sister Judy, one-year-old Jeanne, and I had gone by train from

Mandan to Sauk Centre, Minnesota, to visit my mother's family. It was the first time she'd been back since she and Dennis got married in 1937 and headed west, all their belongings and an out-of-work brother-in-law packed into my dad's truck. During the weeks we were in Minnesota, Dennis wrote two letters to us. One of them began, "Dear Judy and Margie, This is the first time I have the pleasure of writing to my girls." But then the letters stopped. My father never wrote to me again. He never wrote to anyone again. By the time I was five, he was legally blind, unable to drive our Model-A even on the deserted roads around Mandan where he wouldn't meet any traffic except the odd milk truck or hay wagon.

But he had had an earlier life, recorded in the stories he told and the letters he wrote my mother. Those letters are the words of a man who lived by his wits, his strong back, and his eyes. By the time I knew him well, his eyes were all but gone, and his blindness had become the central fact of our lives. Blindness made him think we were endangered, a covey of small girls and a boy on the flat North Dakota prairies. He kept us marooned as he was marooned, trying to guard us from predators and growing, over the years, dark and silent.

People deal with blindness in many ways, and, as I've said, my dad's way was denial, for reasons I've lately begun to probe. Maybe my father's refusal to be and act blind was his protection against the narrow world seeing people imagined for the blind in the forties and fifties, the occupations they trained them for (chair caning, rug making), and the low aspirations they counseled. Maybe he wouldn't accept the vast contrast between what his life had been and what it was fast becoming. He had climbed Mt. Rainier, ridden raw-broken horses, danced till dawn, and then worked a full day threshing grain. Now he should shuffle along with a white cane as conspicuous and bony as an old woman's finger? He might as well sit on the street corner peddling pencils. "You can become anything you want," he told us, and, "Your daddy isn't afraid of anything." In the face of his desperate courage, how could we name the onrushing darkness?

I have seen this blind spot affect my mother and each of us seven kids in a different way. I think we all became a little ashamed, a little more convinced that we were different from most people and not quite normal or respectable. Twice my brother set the hay field near our house on fire, bringing the fire trucks screaming out from town. Lots of boys start fires, and maybe he was just a boy with matches in his pocket and those tempting dry fields; or maybe those near disasters were his flamboyant protest against blindness and the secretiveness that made our lives darker still.

For myself, this secretiveness helped make me a watcher, reading the Braille of bodies, and then a poet, suspicious of surfaces. For if our family hid so momentous a secret from outside eyes, what about all the lives, all the families around us?

I've known the physical facts of my dad's blindness all my life, but because he and I couldn't talk about it, I've had to guess at or imagine the emotional and psychological consequences. What did the physical facts mean, and how did they shape and twist my father's life? How can I know? Through observation and imagination and sympathy, through the knowledge research has given me, and, most recently, through my experience of oncoming blindness. For the blind gene is in me, too, and sooner or later the brightness I see today will fade to gray, then black.

I've read that some people who are born blind and then receive sight are cruelly disappointed by the tattered world that is nowhere near as beautiful as the one they carry in their minds. Dennis Faulkner wasn't born blind; nor did he become blind suddenly, as the result of sickness or an accident. For him there was always

6

dread and always a cruel hope. Along with extreme nearsightedness, he had an inherited disease called "retinitis pigmentosa," a group of diseases that cause the photoreceptor cells in the retina—the rods and cones—to degenerate and eventually die. Because of the name, I used to imagine sullen patches of pigment migrating onto the retina, like green scum moving in from the edge of a pond in the dog days of late August. In reality, the pigmentation is a normal part of the retina. In healthy eyes, an enzyme trims away the pigment; in the eyes of people with RP the enzyme is missing or defective, so the pigment stays put, gradually destroying the cells and narrowing vision on the top, bottom, and sides. Eventually the person is looking out through two tunnels at the milky shapes moving from darkness into darkness. *Light at the end of the tunnel* is a hopeful phrase, promising brighter days ahead, but for the person with RP, tunnels are treacherous and terrifying. He can't trust the air to part magically before him or the ground to lie solid and comforting underfoot. Sidewalks fold and ripple, tripping him. Open cupboard doors leave bruises. Because night blindness usually accompanies RP, my father probably never saw a star. Other dear scenes and faces gradually faded, until all he had was the memory of his children's faces on adolescents and young adults. Researchers haven't determined the exact genetic pathway RP follows in our extended family, and, in fact, we may have inherited two different strains of the disease. While there are exceptions in our family, the general pattern is that fathers pass the disease on to their daughters, most of whom become carriers; the daughters may or may not develop the disease. The daughters can pass the disease on to their sons, with each conception a fifty-fifty flip of the coin; their daughters can also be carriers.

The clichés about blindness, invented to console people for having sight, are partially true at best. I've heard it said hundreds of times that the other senses become keener to compensate for the loss of vision. It's true that my father's ears told him by footstep and voice which one of hundreds of customers had walked into our grocery store and said, "Hello, Faulkner." He played music by ear, on the harmonica, willow whistles, his hands, spoons. He knew meadowlarks and taught us to hear and love their song, knew approaching weather from the sound of the wind and the feel of it on his face. He knew what ailed our 1938 Plymouth from the cough in its motor, and he knew how to fix it. His body and his hands, big, rough, always bruised, became a sea of eyes. Balancing on a one-legged stool, he milked Buttercup, our Jersey cow, his cheek against her warm tan side, milk zinging smartly into the galvanized aluminum pail, the melody changing as the rich milk reached the top. Milking was entirely a matter of feel and rhythm, as was harnessing the big work horses, Ted and Dolly, and hitching them to the plow. But how do you plow a straight furrow if you have no fixed point to help you navigate?

In our image-saturated culture, most of us would do well to close our eyes and call our other senses to life. For all of us, the other senses stir out of their sluggishness when the need arises, guiding us down a black hallway or haltingly down the stairs. But this momentary compensation makes most of us doubly grateful for sight; we realize that for most blind people, blindness is a loss, a lack, the absence of something essential. We have a hard time believing those who call blindness a gift.

But blindness is much more than a matter of physical danger or incapacities.

What is it like to have only footsteps and the thin music of voices? How does dependence, even on loved ones, twist you, making you always angry, a smoldering peat fire easily stirred to flame that blinds your children to your tenderness? What is it like not to be able to see the face of your wife or child crumple in pain when you lash out; not to know if faces are looking at you with pity or amusement, contempt or love; not to see rolled eyes, conspiratorial glances, boredom? What dangers lurk underfoot or to each side, and who's waiting to cheat the old blind guy out of his money, his wife, his kids?

I started working in our grocery story/vegetable market when I was about nine, smart enough to add numbers and make change but no match for two fast-talking con artists. They bought some trifle, then asked me to change a big bill. My dad listened suspiciously, following the transaction in his mind. They left, laughing no doubt, and dad counted the money in the till. We were, as he had suspected, twenty dollars short, a day's profit in 1949.

Dennis was never a man to cater to other people's tastes or opinions. He didn't know or care much about propriety, so even if he hadn't been blind, I doubt that he would have arranged his face to please those around him. But his letters and tender memories show me that he would have worked hard to please the people he loved, that he wouldn't deliberately have hurt them, that the pain on their faces would have been reflected on his. When I was very young, he could still see his children's faces and know if they were sad, happy, or in pain. I often felt loved, held by the tender look on his face and by his velvet voice. I doubt that my youngest sister ever saw that look. By the time she was born, in 1953, my father's eyesight was almost gone. Monie was a blurry shape even when he held her close—soft, warm, with springy curls he could feel, but not with features he could see, find himself in, shape his face to.

After many years of not seeing himself reflected in mirrors, windows, and other faces, I think my dad became invisible to himself. He didn't remember to control the twitches, the bald gestures, the waves of thought and emotion breaking through to the surface. His naked face freed other people to be as thoughtlessly rude as children, who will gaze with fixed, open curiosity at physical disabilities. I watched normally guarded adults watching him, and hated them for their quizzical looks. If he'd been in a wheelchair like President Roosevelt or had had a hook hand or a beautiful red birthmark staining his face, they would have glanced quickly and looked away in embarrassment and compassion. But at my dad with his empty eyes they could look their fill.

By the time I left home for good, Dad often stood at the windows of our grimy little store, staring into the darkness at all hours of the day, his face bitter. He cursed under his breath, not the exuberant, inventive workingman's curses of his earlier years but a bleak, dreary goddamning of his whole life.

Because blindness was an almost untouchable subject in our family, I needed to turn it over in my hands like a family heirloom and do what I've always done: look to the wisdom of the language itself to see what it could teach me about my father's life, my family's life, and mine. I began with the deepest root.

It was a dazzling surprise to find that the Indo-European root of *blind*, thousands of years old, apparently means the opposite, its family as varied and colorful as my mother's flowerbeds. That root—*bhel*—means "to shine, flash, burn; shining white and various bright colors." '*Bhel*' bears on its branches *beluga* and *blush*, as well as *blue* and *flamingo*. It has a branch for *blond*, like my mother and sisters, their pale hair gleaming among the dark-haired German Russians and Bohemians in our hometown. This linguistic tree is a *flamboyant*, so called in Haiti for its blazing umbrella of red-orange blooms. It is a *conflagration* that burns all this brilliance to black, for it bears on one twig the Germanic *blakaz*, "burned"; on another, the old High German *blende*, "to blind, deceive"; and on a third, the Old English *blind*, then as now, verb, noun, adjective, and adverb. The root and trunk of this linguistic tree suggest that there is as much light as there is darkness in being blind.

But the Old English 'blind' apparently fell far from the trunk of its Indo-European tree. In its definitions, synonyms, connotations, and compound forms, there is no color, no refulgence or flamboyance, no playfulness, life, or growth. In the constellation of words surrounding it in the 1992 edition of Roget's *International Thesaurus*, there are only black holes whose inexorable gravity extinguishes all light. In blindness, or so the conventions of the English language say, there is neither light nor germinating darkness. To be blind is to be *closed, drunk, undiscerning, insensible, unaware, unpersuadable, stupid,* or *reckless;* a *blinder* is a pretext, a trick; someone wearing *blinders* is narrow-minded, a *blind story* has no point, and a *blind hedge* has no openings or passages for light.

This linguistic family tree and especially the metaphorical meanings 'blindness' has accumulated over the centuries made me realize that I needed to learn not only about physical blindness but also about all the emotional, intellectual, and spiritual conditions we call by that name. Some of them afflicted my dad; others he resisted. Still others were an unquestioned part of his world. Elizabeth Kelly, my dad's maternal grandmother, brought retinitis pigmentosa with her from Ireland in the steerage compartment of an emigrant ship. That gene or combination of genes has wormed its way silently through the next six generations of our family. I think there's also a communal DNA that follows a twisting path from generation to generation. It manifests itself in our thoughts and actions and our subconscious selves, as well as in family and social patterns. I no longer think it's possible to tell the story of a person or a family without also describing what the Italian cultural theorist Antonio

Gramsci calls the "infinity of traces" history leaves on the psyche of every one of us. As Gramsci says, "It is imperative at the outset to compile . . . an inventory" of history's traces. For my dad wasn't only or even primarily a blind man. For starters, he was a working-class, first-generation Irish American, living in North Dakota in the middle of the twentieth century, a Catholic, a Democrat, a father of six daughters and a son, with each of these historical facts leaving traces on his life. I agree with William Zinsser's assertion in *Inventing the Truth* that "a good memoir is also a work of history, catching a distinctive moment in the life of both a person and a society." I would go further. Good memoirs tell the story of the worlds in which the individual or familial life unfolded and then critique those worlds and their hidden assumptions.

To get to know my father's world I turned to a useful book, *The Chronicle of America*, on the recommendation of poet and memoirist Carolyn Forché. In a memoir writing workshop, she asked us to research the time and place in which our slice of story occurred. I thought this was merely practical advice to help us find historically and geographically authentic details: Who was secretary of state? What songs played incessantly on car radios? What was Senator Joe McCarthy up to? But when I looked up the years 1945, 1947, and 1949, all of which were important to my father's story, I found much more than historical window dressing. I discovered a huge world whose existence I knew about only vaguely or not at all. For instance, I learned that in 1945 hundreds of Japanese Americans were interned at Fort Lincoln, just ten miles east of Mandan. Nineteen forty-seven was the hundredth anniversary of Black '47, the worst year of the Great Famine in Ireland, a disaster all four of my Irish great-grandparents survived. The discoveries kept coming. In 1949 the U.S. government offered the three Indian tribes of Fort Berthold Reservation in northwest North Dakota a few fistfuls of money in exchange for thousands of acres of rich river bottomland. It was an offer they were not free to refuse. In that year, the construction of the Garrison Dam began; when it was completed it would prevent the Missouri River from flooding people like my family who lived downstream. I found other worlds that intersected with ours: the world of the few black people who came into our grocery store in pre–civil rights United States; the world of visually impaired and otherwise disabled people; the world of the Catholic Church of the 1940s and '50s; the patriarchal world with its spoken and unspoken dictates.

So, I set out to trace those big worlds, well aware that historical accounts, too, are full of blind spots, whole blank areas drowned out by the floods of imperialism, colonization, and willed forgetting. Yet part of the work of the memoir is to rescue crucial events from such innocent or deliberate forgetting. As we all know, memory is not made of whole cloth. Gaps in my memory of my dad's life led me to long conversations with my sisters and brother; gaps in history, the story memoirist Patricia Hampl calls "communal memoir," led me to search out immigration records, geography, popular culture, and religion, and to visit museums, graveyards, archives, the old home place. If we didn't know it before, the twentieth century has taught us that nations and ethnic groups, like families, can conspire to forget or deny harsh and ambiguous realities so fiercely that the agreed-upon story, the communal memoir, is either much better or much worse than the real events. That incomplete, distorted, glossed over, romanticized story becomes everyone's memory, the one we print in our history books and pass on to our children. It takes considerable searching, then, to unearth and tell a more complex and often more painful version. Still, as honest scholars admit, some information is lost forever. I hope the gaps and holes in my account will pull others into the conversation—in agreement, disagreement, correction, expansion—as I explore blindness in its many physical and cultural permutations.

TWO

Blinders

Leather flaps on a bridle, to prevent a horse from
seeing sideways. Fig., obstacles to clear judgment
or perception.

I F YOU DON'T HAVE THE shiny icons of a prosperous life, you
can be blinded temporarily or permanently to what your life
does have–its homeliness, its friendly intimacy, its shelter-
ing curves and inviting spaces, its sensual richness. Though my
father worked as hard as he could all his life, our family was
never more than a step or two ahead of poverty. When he died
at seventy, my mother couldn't scrape up enough money for his
coffin and had to pay for it on installments.

We didn't have indoor plumbing when I was growing up. We
had an outdoor toilet, freezing in winter, stifling and fly infested
in summer, with crinkly pink peach wrappers or the soft index
sheets from Sears catalogs for toilet paper. Until I learned to
be ashamed and even after, I didn't hate that toilet, or, as my
mother called it, "the can." On cold winter nights, before my

five sisters and I crawled into bed, we piled into the toilet. There were two seats, a high one with an adult-sized hole and a low one for short legs and little bottoms. We told stories out there while we waited for the little kids to finish their business; after we acquired a flashlight, we terrified ourselves by shining it straight up and bringing a hand down over the light, a giant claw descending.

Our bathtub was a galvanized aluminum wash tub as round as a moon that grew tighter and tighter as we grew to womanhood and manhood. In the summer my mother filled it with brownish yellow rainwater caught in the wooden barrel on the cool north-west corner of the house. In winter we smelled the metallic tang of snow melting all day Saturday in the tub on the oil-burning heater. Every Saturday night until each of us went off to college, we bathed in that tub, youngest to oldest, with my mother and father bringing up the rear and finally emptying the water on the snow or on some patch of grass that welcomed water of any kind in the dry North Dakota summers. While we bathed we listened to the nasal twang of the *Grand Ol' Opry.* Until I learned better, I loved the songs, especially Hank Williams' remarkably similar renderings of "The Old Rugged Cross" and "Old Shep Was a Dog," both of which made me cry.

As I think back on that cramped little house and the life that necessarily spilled out into the yard and gardens and surrounding fields, I hear angry words and tears tangled with laughter and songs and an endless supply of stories, most of which we made up on the fly. There was a lot of work to do, and all of us kids had to help with it; but both Mom and Dad encouraged us to sing while we did the piles of dishes and make up dramas as we worked in the garden, declaring war on the creeping jenny and quack grass, whose roots surely reached to the center of the earth. Our mission was to kill "the wild jenny weed," hacking at it viciously with hoes.

BLINDERS

While the town kids joined Boy Scouts and Girl Scouts, went to Saturday matinees at the Mandan theater, and swam in the town pool, we had Sunday afternoon picnics under the Big Tree, an old cottonwood that rustled secretively all summer and in fall dropped tough yellow leaves that we braided into long chains. Though none of us knew how to swim, we went down to a channel of the Heart River, with its dangerous currents, drop-offs, and quicksand, and rode big logs and a raft we built and named "Old Drifter." Amazingly, no one drowned or got seriously hurt; we were protected, Mom often said, by her fervent prayers to our guardian angels.

What we couldn't afford, we improvised. Ballet lessons weren't even a dream, so Judy permanently borrowed a book from the school library, and from looking at the pictures, we learned foot and hand positions and a cockeyed version of turns, leaps, and arabesques that we performed in the yard. We put on circuses, Christmas pageants, and our own costume parties every Halloween.

We jumped double Dutch, making up our own rhymes when we got tired of the ones we learned in school, played baseball with three or four players to a side, at least two of whom were there under weekly duress, and shot cans off the fence with Dennie's BB gun. We couldn't afford bikes, and, anyway, Highway 10 was too dangerous to ride on. Instead, we had roller skates on which we made endless noisy circles around the counter in Dad's store. We rode into the Wild West on our teeter-totter—a wide plank over a saw horse with a blanket for a saddle and a rope for reins. Most of all, we made up stories, endless stories with characters and dialogue borrowed from radio shows. (We didn't get a TV until I was fifteen, so the images of Tom Mix, the Lone Ranger, and Hopalong Cassidy were our own.)

This seems at first like a childhood I'd want for all children. We were free from scheduled play and too much adult supervision. Our imaginations were fertile and unfettered and fed by Dad's stories and songs. We loved it when he cupped his harmonica in his big rough hands and played a mournful or a jaunty song. My sister Jeanne described in a poem what those songs did for us:

> My father's harmonica
> cried, crooned, and cajoled us
> with the haunting tales
> of wayward winds and valleys low.
> My father's harmonica
> laughed loudly, lyrically
> about Irish washer women.
> Dancing on worn wooden floors
> we forgot the handouts,
> the hunger for what he
> could never give.
> My father's harmonica
> wailed, wooed, and whistled,
> freeing our hearts from wishing.

But a family can be both strong and fragile at the same time, and there were times when the music and the make-believe were no shelter at all, at least for me. For no matter how isolated or protected a family is, it never fully resists the influence of the surrounding worlds; like every person, a family bears the traces of its history. This was Mandan, North Dakota, in the thirties, forties, and fifties. It wasn't a place of grace and elegance, and it's likely that many of our classmates at St. Joseph's Grade School and Mandan High School grew up in homes as small and crowded as ours. But I never risked finding out. I learned very young to hide the shabbiness of our lives from most outsiders. I also learned early to believe that anything that made us different made us less. If blindness was a shameful thing, how much more a smelly toilet and a bathtub most people had seen only in caricature on funny post cards? This was how the Okies lived, the hillbillies, the poor people my mother had us pray for every night after we had God-blessed Grandma and asked God to cure our daddy's eyes. The only recourse was to pass for middle class by day and protect the life of our family from prying eyes. Because we lived so far from my parents' families, and most of our relatives had no money for travel, we rarely had visitors. When they did come, we kids were delighted, but I can imagine my mother's humiliation in pointing her sister-in-law with the blue-white hair and the genteel job at Penney's toward the outdoor toilet and the enamel washbasin in the kitchen, grimy with hard-water scum no matter how often Mom scrubbed it.

A few years ago, I met a young African American writer who told me that she used to gaze hungrily at the pictures of families in her school hygiene book—a mother, father, and two children eating food separated into isolated portions of the plate, a pork chop on one side, potatoes nearby but not quite touching the chop or the neat pile of peas. If her family could eat like that, then they'd be like that, and they'd belong. But her family, made up of her mother, grandmother, grandfather, and her, ate greasy slabs of cornbread pie that covered the plate.

I yearned, too, for a long white bathtub I could point out nonchalantly to my friends and a lawn as flat and green as paint like the ones in our Dick and Jane book, instead of the cracked, gray river-bottom soil and the weeds, some of them taller than I was, that filled our yard.

Our mother, a wonderful seamstress, sent us to school clean and starched in dresses made of flour sacks and recycled rummage-sale garments. Every day she curled our hair around her finger and polished our shoes. One day, late in first grade, she taught me an unforgettable lesson. When I came home from school that day, I told my mother what had happened and who had said what, as I always did. "Becky asked me why I always wear the same dress and I told her I only have two and the other one is in the wash."

Mom's blue eyes got round with shock. "Oh no! Never tell anybody that. You should have said you wear it because you like it."

Now I was shocked, but not because my mother, who always asked for the truth, was telling me to lie. By then I knew the usefulness of lies. You lied to protect yourself from your parents' anger and sometimes to protect them from some piece of information that might hurt them. But why did my clothes need protection? What was wrong with having only two dresses? I did like them, that was true. The one I was wearing that day had tiny blue and white checks, and my mother had made it beautiful by attaching white rickrack to the collar with red hemstitching as delicate as lace. The white checks and collar shone with cleanliness.

But if its lowly beginnings as a flour sack and the fact that it had only one companion on the broomstick behind the curtain that was our closet were shameful enough to need the camouflage of lies, what else in my home and my family needed protection? My mother obviously knew about some danger I had missed. I know now that she was trying to protect me from the scorn of my richer classmates, but the lesson I learned was no protection at all.

I didn't blame her then and don't blame her now. She had felt what Tillie Olsen calls "the hidden injuries of class." For fifteen years, from the time she left school after eighth grade until she married my father at age twenty-seven, she worked as a maid for doctors' families in Sauk Centre, Minnesota. The doctors' wives and daughters never let her forget that she was a servant. Early in her marriage, when the Great Depression still hung over North Dakota, the person we called "the welfare woman" stopped by now and then, especially after spring floods, bringing food and those precious flour sacks. We kids found her entertaining, but I have only recently tried to imagine what it was like for my mother and father, hard working, farm raised, having supported themselves and their families from childhood, to have to accept charity.

I remember the time in first grade when I wanted a medallion so badly my stomach ached for it. It was maroon glass with a filigree gold cover that opened up, and it hung on a golden chain. Inside was a small rosary the same color as the case. It was holy and beautiful and cost a dollar. All the girls bought them, or at least all the girls I considered rich. I don't remember begging my mother for that dollar, just shyly describing the medallion's unearthly beauty and asking her if I could get one. In 1946 a dollar bought four pounds of hamburger, enough for two meals if my mother stretched it. A dollar for a first-grader's necklace was a reckless expense. Still, seeing my yearning, my mother saved the money somehow, but by the time she handed it to me, the medallions were all gone. How sad and disappointed was she for me, her quiet daughter who was born blue and hairless and almost died? Did all of our disappointments roll up into a huge load that she shouldered every day, as she tried to keep the world from falling on each of her seven children?

And what about my dad? Did the weight of our poverty rest even more heavily on him? His letters to my mom suggest that it did. He was about forty-one or forty-two when he wrote those letters; in them, longing for marriage and family and his and Hattie's work are equally important because they depend on each other. On August 24, 1937, just three months before he and Hattie got married, he apologized for one more delay:

I didn't blame you for getting impatient I am myself but a good friend of mine told me yesterday that if I waited to get rich before I got married I would have to wait a long time. But I have always worried if we were married and I didn't have lots of money you would get disgusted and leave me. And the lord knows I would much rather stay single than for that to happen. I know two men who had to send their wives home to their folks this summer. Well if I had to do that I would be so ashamed I couldn't look at anybody. So honey you can't blame me for worrying and trying to make good.

To "get rich" enough to marry my mother Dennis baled tons of alfalfa in 108-degree heat, helped build a state highway, worked at Swift's meat-packing plant, and traveled all over two states working or looking for work. Most working men were hard up, and the competition for jobs was stiff. He had to go where the work was. His working days were often twelve hours or longer, and his weeks seven days, with an hour off for church. He talked about being rich enough to marry, but his notion of riches was touchingly modest, and at the time most people's prospects were often desperate. In one letter he wrote that his younger brother Bill—twenty-six years old, over six feet tall, strong and used to hard work—threshed grain for $2.50 a day.

Dennis's luck turned, or so he thought, just a month before his marriage, when he rented a big vegetable stand on Highway 10, between Bismarck and Mandan. He sold vegetables that Bill hauled from the Red River Valley two hundred miles to the east. In a letter that sounds almost jubilant, he wrote to Hattie: "I am here all alone and a steady go from morning til 12 at night. . . . I think I have taken in $25.00 already today and its only 3:30 and over $40.00 yesterday." This is the place he brought Hattie to, right after they got married on October 26, 1937. We grew up there and eventually left it behind.

Predictably, we children fled the smells and sounds and sights of our home, each in our own way. My older sister Judy, feeling the most trapped and the most misplaced of us all, got as far away from Mandan and that Nashville twang as she could go, even while she was still at home. In the face of universal ridicule, every Saturday afternoon she listened to the Texaco Opera broadcast from the Met. "La Dona è mobile" and "Vesti la giuba" sailed on waves of heat in our little kitchen as Judy helped with the week's baking. All of us fled into books and finally to college. Can our parents have guessed that education would take their children away from them in that familiar American good-luck-story way? Can they have guessed that our books would label and classify them and the life they'd made for us? My father must have sensed some such danger. By the force of his personality and his fatherly authority, he tried to keep us marooned as he was marooned in a world that year by year grew tighter and more confining.

In the books that became my life's work, I eventually found a word to describe the ways in which he exerted his authority over his family. I hadn't been studying women, their lives, and their writing long before I came upon the word *patriarchy*, the rule by the fathers, and *patriarch*, the father who rules the family, the church, the state. I immediately recognized our dad. In our house, there could be no question about whose word was law. Mom had amazing strength, resourcefulness, intelligence, and practical creativity; she worked alongside Dad from morning until night and knew as much as he did about every angle of our precarious livelihood. Yet she had to ask him for permission to go into town and for money to spend, not on frills but on necessities. She rarely challenged his decisions, at least not in front of us kids.

I remember only two occasions when she took a stand and stuck to it. The first was the time she bought a couple of swimming suits and drove us to the swimming lessons we'd been begging for all summer. The second brave stand changed our lives forever. When Judy, the oldest, was eighteen and ready for college, Mom borrowed against the life insurance policy she'd been paying into for thirty years. She got only four hundred dollars, but it was enough to pay Judy's first-year tuition at the College of St. Benedict in St. Joseph, Minnesota, a world away from Mandan. The rest of us eventually followed, always over Dad's objections. Like many Irish American fathers, he thought daughters as well as sons needed an education, in case they never married or a dead, drunk, or runaway husband made them the breadwinners for the family. "Learn all you can, girls," he used to tell us. "It's the only thing they can't take away from you." But he had something practical in mind, accounting and bookkeeping, leading to a steady job in a bank, or maybe nursing, so we could be like his Aunt Maggie Maloney; she was "a professional nurse," as her father's obituary says, who came home to the farm in Leaf Valley, Minnesota, to tend him in his last illness. When I was a senior in high school, I turned down a secure job as secretary to our high school superintendent and followed Judy to St. Ben's to study English. My dad urged me to take the secretarial job, and I'm sure it was only my mother's and my sister's courage that made me brave enough to go against his wishes.

But my mother's acts of rebellion were rare. Most of the time, Dad was the breadwinner, the keeper of the purse, the final decision maker. Though he often said to us, "Kids, you've got the best mom in the world," he sometimes ignored Mom's wishes in shocking ways. One whole winter he kept a glass-topped cage of rattlesnakes by the front door of our store, given to him by a bounty hunter who apparently caught rattlers for a living. Mom was terrified of all snakes, considering them the devil incarnate, and begged him to get rid of them. He laughed at her fears, assuring her that the cage was escape-proof, and showed off the snakes to the men who came to our store. Finally, the big 1952 flood carried away the cage and its whirring inhabitants, no doubt to the horror of someone downriver.

Though Mom had to ask for money, Dad sometimes gave her presents that were lavish, at least by our standards. The one I remember best was a long, quilted taffeta lounge robe. It was reversible, royal blue on one side, deep rose on the other. I'm certain he offered the robe as a sign of his love but also as evidence of his ability to provide more than a bare-bones life for her. But it was a shocking waste of money in a house with no bathroom for a woman who never had time to lounge. The robe stayed in its box most of the time, except for a rare hour after Mom's Saturday night bath when my sisters and I gathered on her bed to give each other manicures or when it became the Blessed Virgin's robe in our Christmas plays.

Dad's shifting moods also ruled our lives. He had a ready though unpredictable sense of humor. One summer day when we were very young, Mom had set the week's supply of bread to rise in the hot kitchen while she worked in the garden. We were supposed to be napping, but those round, white bellies of bread were irresistible. When Mom came in, hot and tired with supper still to make, she found ten grubby finger holes in every deflated loaf. I went outside, knowing that the yard was a much safer place than the kitchen. Around the corner I came upon Dad, laughing so hard tears ran down his cheeks. He knew that our mischief meant more work for Mom, as it always did. He didn't want her to hear him laughing, but the sight of those loaves—the handiwork of his little daughters—cracked him up. But his moods were volatile, and on another day, a similarly inventive experiment would have made him very angry. We kids disobeyed our dad at our peril, risking his anger and threats of abandonment, which I now know he would never have carried out. But when I was a child, I believed him. I could usually predict when he would get mad at my older sister Judy for some small misdeed and threaten to take her to the girls' reform school in Mandan where, we had heard, girls' heads were shaved as they were in German concentration camps. I begged my beloved sister to say she was sorry, give in, do whatever he told her to do. She raged back at him, and the rest of us did all the giving in.

We once had a gray work horse named Ted who spent most of his life harnessed to a plow, disk, harrow, or hay wagon, pulling with Dolly, his partner. He was a hard worker when he was in harness, his eyes shielded with blinders. Without the blinders, he was a runaway, who regularly jumped over a low place in the fence and headed for the far horizon. We'd get into the Model A and drive down country roads looking for him. There he'd be, grazing peacefully in a road ditch or in someone else's pasture. My dad would tie him to the car's bumper and lead him home.

Like Ted's blinders, patriarchal injunctions have kept both women and men doggedly plowing dusty furrows marked out for them in countless cultures through countless centuries. These injunctions blind parents to their own far-flung talents, yearnings, and needs and to those of their sons and daughters. They guided Mom's actions as well as Dad's and were, oddly, most damaging for Dennie, the only boy in a crowd of girls. My mom fretted about the proper way to raise a son. Above all, she didn't want to coddle him and turn him into a sissy. Dennie remembers when she stopped tucking him into bed when he was very small. He can remember her strong, cool, tender hands from that last time. Then the tenderness stopped, and he thought, This is how it's going to be for me from now on. But he was still his dad's buddy, until that, too, changed.

For the first six or seven years of his life, Dennie was the prince, the namesake, the longed-for son after four daughters. He and Dad were companions and friends. Like many little boys, Dennie adored our dad and wanted to be just like him: strong, tall, confident, a storyteller with a big, rowdy laugh. When Dennie was about ten, everything changed. He felt as if our dad abandoned him, and instead of being a prince, he became a stupid person who would never amount to anything, a damn girl who should be in the house wearing a dress, not outside among men doing men's work. Worst of all, he felt alone, with no one to lean on and no hand to hold. Instead of being my dad's best buddy, Dennie became his reluctant guide, the arm Dad held on his rare trips into town. This shift that seemed so sudden followed Dad's slide into blindness and silence and his loss of confidence in himself as the strong, sure head of the family. From this distance, it seems as if the harsh words he flung at his son were really meant for himself.

I've read several memoirs and autobiographies by men who lost their sight. Almost all of them have had to come to terms sooner or later with the ways in which blindness threatens their sense of themselves as men. Of course, every blind person has to face her or his dependency over and over in the big and small affairs of everyday life, a dependency that well-meaning sighted friends, family members, and strangers often make more humiliating by reducing the blind person to the status of a child. While dependency isn't easy for anyone (think of all the three-year-olds who assert, "I can do it my own self"), it must be more demeaning for men than for women in a culture where independence, strength, and the ability to support and defend women and children are part of the very definition of manhood.

John Hull became blind at forty-five after the birth of his second child. He and his wife had three more children in the next few years. In *Touching the Rock*, his journal of the three years from 1983 to 1986, when he was trying to make sense of his blindness, he wrote honestly and painfully about his life as a husband and father, as a man. He says, for example, "A disabled adult man loses part of his manhood, part of his adulthood, and part of his humanity. I know Jesus told us we should repent and become as little children, but I don't want it in this way. I don't like having my adulthood wrenched from me like this." He wrote even more movingly about feeling "marginalized as a father," shut out of his children's games, "impotent, unable to survey, to admire, or to exercise jurisdiction or discrimination." He wrote about how he learned to enter his son's "birthday world," but he called that chapter "Lost Children," suggesting that in some ways his children's world would always be closed to him. On a visit with his family to Australia where he was born and grew up, he felt keenly the difference between his old self and his new blind self. Though this transformation had many dimensions, one of the most painful was the reduction of his role as father and leader of his family: "I still have difficulty in renouncing my role as father, as the convivial one who always makes others feel at home. How can I any longer count on being reliable in good company? How can I any longer take the initiative in anecdotes and witticisms? What about my role as leader and guide to my own children? I am sharply conscious of the difficulty of showing the place off to them. . . . I cannot even point out the strange animals to the children unless I get a description first of what they look like."

My father wasn't a writer like John Hull and didn't have the words to describe what it was like to be relegated to the edges of his children's lives as we ran to him on Christmas morning to show him toys he couldn't see, balls he couldn't catch, or books he couldn't read to us.

In an old picture of my dad, one of the rare ones in which he's smiling, he's holding Judy, the first baby, in one arm. In the other hand he's holding a brace of pheasants. He wouldn't have taken credit for another man's game, so he must still have been able to see well enough to sight along the gray barrel of the shotgun and follow the birds as they flew up from the fields. By the time his only son was ready to handle a gun, Dad couldn't have seen a bear lumbering toward him. There were no father-son hunting adventures, and Dennie taught himself to shoot. Eventually, all seven of us turned away, looking elsewhere for wisdom, knowledge, and practical advice, even though Dad had rich stores of all three that he would have given to us gladly if we could have found a way to break through the silence.

Eric Weihenmayer's memoir, *Touching the Top of the World*, contains some of the most revealing comments I've found about the perceived relationship between sight and masculinity. He's one of only a hundred people in the history of the world who have climbed the highest mountain peak on every continent. He's been blind since age fifteen, began rock climbing at sixteen, and by thirty-three had performed the amazing feat of scaling Mount Everest. You wouldn't think he'd have any doubts about his manhood. Faced with twenty-five-thousand feet of mountain, Weihenmayer is respectful, quietly confident, and humble. As he says, "That is what I like about mountains. It is a realm where humans haven't reached godlike status, a realm that demands humility." Faced with women, on the other hand, Weihenmayer's respect, confidence, and humility seem to desert him. As a teenager he got his first taste of rock climbing at Carroll Center for the Blind in Massachusetts. He also got a taste of the hierarchy created even by partial sight. The "Partials" were able to lead the "Totals," and all the girls wanted to be with the partially blind boys. Weihenmayer writes that "testosterone levels were linked in some way to [the boys'] level of vision. How much they could see became a fierce competition." He admits that he, like the other campers, "bought into the subtle message that sight meant power." And, I would add, sight meant masculine prowess.

As an adult, in his dealings with women, Weihenmayer boasts: "Some people think that blind people do not care about looks, that we are above assessing one's desirability through surface beauty, but if that's the case, I proudly break the stereotype. I am as much a pig as any sighted guy. In fact, I take offense at those who would assume that just because I am blind I am supposed to be asexual. Blindness has little to do with the virtue or villainy of one's character. I can be just as shallow, but my shallowness comes from the voluptuous hum of a sexy voice or the electrifying grasp of a smooth supple hand." Weihenmayer works out a system of handshakes and under-the-table kicks with his sighted friends so that he doesn't get stuck with a woman whose face and figure aren't as beautiful and voluptuous as her voice. What's most shocking about this comment is that it comes right after Weihenmayer as teacher states his determination to "remain blissfully ignorant," getting to know his fifth-grade students as "charming, innocent, young people with promise and intelligence" rather than as the "chubby, unfashionable nose pickers" the other teachers insist upon describing to him.

I certainly don't think blind men are asexual, nor do I expect them to be any more or less virtuous than the general run of human beings, simply because they are blind. But it saddens me that this smart, brave, imaginative young man, writing in the twenty-first century, can't imagine his way past the stereotype of manhood that gives him the right to turn women into objects he judges and weighs, sometimes literally. (Once he tricked his fiancée into stepping onto his talking scale, whose robotic voice obediently revealed her weight to him.) His comments also help me understand my dad, who lived at a time when almost no one questioned gender stereotypes. As his life became narrower and darker, his sense of himself as a man who could hold his own among men seems to have gradually eroded, worn away by his struggles to support his family and by his deepening blindness.

Of course, we never talked about the painful subject of Dad's loss of self-confidence, but I can guess at some of the causes, helped by the insights of other men who went blind later in life. Robert Hine a college history professor who became totally blind at fifty after a long decline, writes: "It worried me that sightlessness was also blinding me to [my wife's] needs. Did she ever crave a man who was more protective, who could recognize danger a mile away, who could instantly rise to stand between her and harm?"

Dad, who worried about everything, must have felt a similar uneasiness. I remember two contrasting incidents. One Sunday we came home from church to find the front window of our store broken and Dad massaging his right hand in a friendly way, a pleased little smile on his face. He told us the story with quiet pride and none of the usual ornamentation: a drunk came in demanding liquor. When Dad refused and told him to hit the road, the man foolishly got belligerent. With one well-placed uppercut, Dad put him through the window. On a rainy night not long after, Dad was outside the store filling a woman's gas tank, while she was inside emptying the cash drawer. Of course, this could happen to anyone. People steal from sighted people all the time. But Dad cried when he told us what had happened, for the loss of the money, which we always needed badly, but even more for the loss of his confidence, his fearlessness, and his ability to protect those entrusted to him. "It's all gone," he said. These worries might explain his jealousy, a period of several years when he drank heavily, his increasing silence and smoldering anger, his overprotectiveness that often felt both smothering and illusory, and his apparent abandonment of his only son.

Even though my dad seems to fit smoothly into the definition of patriarchy and the version of manhood that was only too familiar in the forties and fifties, he did not have a secure place in the hierarchy of wealth, power, and status. For a man like my father, a generic label such as *patriarch* can also become a set of blinders for sons and daughters who miss the far horizons of their fathers' lives because they see them plowing only that one stubborn furrow.

From the time I was very young, I knew that my dad wasn't the kind of man I read about in my books or occasionally saw in my friends' houses. Those men wore suits and ties, and their day jobs as doctors or owners of the creamery, the shoe store, or the bank conferred status; they were powerful, wealthy, and distant, living in a separate world from their wives and children. Nor was our dad like the railroad men or mechanics who left early in the morning and came home just at suppertime, after a stop at the Silver Dollar for a snort or two.

First of all, Dad didn't look the part. To save money, he had haircuts as seldom as possible, waiting until his bushy gray hair reached his collar. He wore work clothes except for one hour on Sunday. Because our store and garden were a few yards from our house, he was always home and ate breakfast, dinner, and supper with us. In fact, traditional male and female roles often blurred in the way my parents, by necessity, divided up the work. My mom did the driving, wrote the checks and balanced the checkbook, made out orders for fireworks and produce, and kept records. While Dad didn't wash dishes, make beds, or do laundry, he dressed and fed the little kids and helped Mom cut cabbage for huge crocks of sauerkraut. Once he even tried to shell peas for canning by putting them through the washing machine wringer. This labor-saving plan failed, and soon peas were shooting all over the kitchen, and Mom and Dad were bent over laughing. Dad was involved in his kids' learning, often much too involved for our happiness, as he drilled us on multiplication tables we couldn't master (he called it "rapid calculation") or words we couldn't spell. (For some reason, *paraphernalia* was one of his favorite stumpers.)

In an era and place when men were supposed to be stoic, he was openly emotional, easily moved to tenderness and even tears in response to other people's suffering, especially the suffering of children. His letters to my mom are filled with honest confessions of feeling: lonesomeness, a shy happiness when she agreed to marry him, and compassion for his sister Clara when her baby died and for an illegitimate nephew who nobody seemed to know what to do with. He wrote, "If we were married we could take the little boy. Well there could be nothing that would please me more than that." And in another letter, he said, "The way I feel I would do anything before I would see him go to strangers." He brought that tenderness into the early years of marriage and fatherhood. In 1942, when Mom and the first three kids were in Minnesota for several weeks visiting relatives, he wrote frequent letters. In one of them he said: "I am fine only when I see something of yours or the little girls play things the tears just won't stop running but sweetheart don't worry. I'll be alright no matter how long you are away for my heart is down there with [you] all the time."

His tenderness was often obscured by his quick, unpredictable temper and his constant worry over money. But when I search my memories of him, I see him holding Rocky, our friendly black and white dog. Rocky ran free as all our dogs did, chasing cars and snuffing at rabbits in the pasture but always coming home for a supper of table scraps and a bed under the porch. One day he got into a brutal fight with the German shepherd who guarded the El Rancho nightclub right next door. Rocky got the worst of the fight. A few days later, the day I remember, the right side of Rocky's head was swollen to twice its size, his eye closed, and the wound red and dangerous looking. He put his head on Dad's lap and whimpered. A trip to the vet was out of the question; we didn't even go to the doctor for human injuries. So Mom and Dad became the doctors. Dad held Rocky's head and washed the wound, and Mom poured peroxide straight from the bottle. Rocky struggled, then held still. Dad said, "He knows we're trying to help him." Rocky's wound healed, and he lived to chase many more cars until one day he didn't dodge fast enough and a car hit and killed him. It happened during the day, when we were all at school. When we came home, and Rocky didn't run to meet us, Mom and Dad said that he must be chasing rabbits in the woods. He'd be back. Of course, he never came back, but it was years before they told us that our happy dog had been killed.

We kids were used to death and unsentimental about it. Rocky's four predecessors had also been killed on the highway. Whole litters of kittens died of distemper, and after a proper burial, we turned to the next litter. When we were very young, Mom often killed an old hen for Sunday dinner with one shining down-swing of the hatchet. We watched with delight as the headless chicken flapped wildly around the yard, its jugular spurting blood. Then we stood around the kitchen table, our noses barely clearing the edge, and watched Mom clean the hen, her strong, blue-veined hands pulling out red and purple guts, rich yellow fat, and, sometimes, the treasure of a thin-shelled egg, even a double-yoker. I don't remember being shocked or disgusted or deeply grieved by any of these deaths. Like most country kids, we took them in stride. But Rocky was different. Dad and Mom knew it and agreed to spare their children the sadness of his death.

I often saw Dad unmanned, that strangely powerful word that describes a ship sailing with no one at the rudder, left to the forces of nature, or a spaceship in the outer reaches of the universe where it's too dangerous or rarified to send a human being—or a man overcome by his feelings. He cried when Coreen came home from the eye doctor year after year with the same ominous verdict: her eyes hadn't improved; when his mother died; when he came to my profession ceremony as a Benedictine sister and heard the snip of the scissors cutting my hair, a ritual he couldn't see and certainly couldn't understand or accept. But because being unmanned implies a dangerous weakness, he often belied his tender side by courting danger; telling bold, memorable stories; and singing Woody Guthrie songs from the Great Depression that were equal parts lament, brag, and protest: "The Biggest Thing That Man Has Ever Done," "Lonesome Road Blues," "We Ain't Down Yet." Sometimes he played harmonica riffs between the verses. So Dad both was and wasn't a patriarch, his grip on manhood compromised by his lowly place on the economic ladder, by his personality, and by his blindness. Men whose manhood is threatened in the worlds of work and social power often try to reclaim it in the intimate relationships of marriage and family. Wives, sons, and daughters are then called to the painful task of balancing love, anger, and resistance. I think it's impossible for most kids to hang on to these contradictory feelings. Either we love our domineering fathers and obey with or without questioning, or we rebel against fatherly authority that seems unjust and arbitrary and refuse the trap of love. The losses are great no matter which choice a child makes, often before she knows she's making it.

I don't want to speak for my sisters and brother but only for myself. As far back as I can remember, I loved Dad deeply and painfully, feeling more sympathy for him than a child should feel for her father; because of that love and sympathy, I almost lost my ability to question, challenge, and act independently. When college offered me the chance, I went away, as we all did. After college I had many reasons for deciding to become a Benedictine sister, another choice that bewildered and saddened my dad. A reason I admitted to myself only recently is that I didn't want a marriage like my parents'. I was afraid my newly formed ideas and convictions, seedlings with tentative roots, would wither. Later still, taught in part by my rebellious high school students chanting, "I am woman, hear me roar!" I learned to question all patriarchal authority, including my dad's. But I was lucky. I entered the women's movement through the writing of Tillie Olsen, Grace Paley, and Meridel LeSueur, writers of the working class whose stories encouraged me to see in a clear, unwavering, but sympathetic light my father and working men like him. These stories also encouraged me to take another look at the life I left behind in Mandan. I don't want to romanticize it; there was nothing quaint or chosen about our version of simple living. But there was a lot that was honest and rich and true.

In spite of the hierarchy in our family, my parents were a matched team, pulling together, with their eyes on the same horizon. They wanted to keep their children healthy and safe and make a better life for them—a life in which none of their six daughters would be maids in the homes of the well-to-do, and their son would not have to wander the country looking for work and wondering whether he'd ever have a secure job with a living wage so he could support a family. To make this better life possible, Mom and Dad were willing to "share want" with each other, to borrow another of Tillie Olsen's powerful phrases. They didn't want to be rich, nor did they burden us with such expectations. Mom's classic question was, "They're rich, but are they happy?" And though Dad worked hard all his life and bent and broke the law to make enough money to support his family, he never wanted lots of possessions or a big bankroll. In fact, he mistrusted and even despised rich people, sometimes repeating a funny saying he must have learned from his Irish clan or from his fellow organizers in the Nonpartisan League: "The devil always shits on the biggest pile," implying, of course, that there's no way to amass a pile of money without making a dirty deal with the devil.

In place of a desire for wealth, Dad and Mom gave us a life where beauty and whimsy were almost as important as food and clean clothes, though I don't remember either of them ever talking about such a notion. Mom's hands spoke for her, beautifying everything they touched. She dried rough cotton sheets in the sun and wind and ironed them as smooth as fine percale. She raised a flamboyant array of flowers that appeared in jelly glasses in every room of our house. Our pretty dresses were much more than a camouflage for poverty. Even if no one outside our family had ever seen them, she would have made them with the same care and the same sure eye for color and line. I can see her now, the year I was seven, making herself a new Sunday dress, one of only two she had while we were growing up. It was of brown rayon, with a mermaid tail down the side. We gathered around her, my sisters and I, and watched her create a peacock of sequins, stitch by stitch. It was red and green and turquoise with one gold eye, and it perched on her shoulder and spread its tail across our lives. With a length of cloth and a bead or two, she made our ramshackle life bloom. One of Dad's money-making schemes was raising gladiolus to cut and sell in bouquets. As I recall, this venture was a lot of work, and we never sold many flowers. But when I shut my eyes I can still see in my mother's flower bed row upon row of lavender, peach, and fuchsia flowers on slender green stems. Dad taught us to love meadowlarks and music, rhythm and dance, books, stories, and the power of language to create worlds much bigger and more fantastic than the one we lived in.

In spite of our isolation on the outskirts of Mandan, our parents taught us to renounce individualism in favor of responsibility for others. Mom and Dad never turned away the ragged men who jumped off the freight trains that passed within a few hundred yards of our house. We didn't call these men "transients," "migrants," or "hoboes"; those names were too fancy. They were "tramps" or "bums," hungry and needing a handout. Because of my parents' frugality and hard work, they always had something to give—a sandwich, a bunch of overripe bananas—and because of their largeness of soul, they were somehow sure there'd still be enough for the family. Even that taffeta bathrobe was a lesson in lavish giving: every now and then throw money over your shoulder so that it doesn't own you. By their lives, both Mom and Dad taught us to question conventional standards of beauty, goodness, success, and happiness, making all seven of us awkward tenants in mainstream U.S.A.

I agree with poet Mary Oliver, who says, "In this universe we are given two gifts: the ability to love and the ability to question. Which are, at the same time, the fires that warm us and the fires that scorch us." As I said earlier, children have a hard time holding on to these apparently contradictory impulses. Maybe one of the good, painful uses of memory is to return to our pasts—our parents, families, homes—and, denying neither the harm done nor the gifts given and received, see them in the light cast by those two fires.

THREE

Blind

Out of sight, out of the way, secret, obscure

BECAUSE BLINDNESS WAS our family secret, and because I distanced myself from it as steadfastly as my dad did, I never learned much about it, though my mind and feelings were always secretly attuned. Until I began to do research for this book, I'd never even read Helen Keller's autobiography, though I'd laughed uneasily at my share of Helen Keller jokes. Studying the history of blindness in the United States, watching the portrayal of men and women who are blind in the mainstream media, and reading autobiographies and memoirs helped me to understand my dad's anger and depression, his recklessness and courage, and his stubborn refusal to acknowledge his blindness and learn adaptive techniques. I learned that he wasn't as alone in these reactions as I'd thought. I also learned that the category of people lumped together and labeled *the blind* doesn't exist in reality. Like all handy labels, this one has a way of growing until it eclipses the array of people it claims to describe, sometimes becoming their whole identity, in the minds and eyes of those around them and, worse yet, in their own minds. Robert Hine says that during his fifteen years of blindness, "I found it easy sometimes to identify myself with my disability. I was not a man; I was a blind man. I was not a professor; I was a blind professor."

In Toni Morrison's novel *Song of Solomon,* wise old Pilate, who sees what's hidden, says:

You think dark is just one color, but it ain't. They're five or six kinds of black. Some silky, some woolly. Some just empty. Some like fingers. And it don't stay still. It moves and changes from one kind of black to another. Saying something is pitch black is like saying something is green. What kind of green? Green like my bottles? Green like a grasshopper? Green like a cucumber, lettuce, or green like the sky is just before it breaks loose to storm? Well, night black is the same way. May as well be a rainbow.

For profound physical, psychological, and social reasons, blindness isn't all one color either. People who are blind are as different from each other as people who can see, having in common just that one characteristic. I'm ashamed to say that this diversity surprised me. I don't want to assume that everyone is as unaware of the wildly varied experiences of blindness as I was. Still, the ways in which blindness is construed in our language, our media, our schools, and especially our workplaces tells me that the generic label *the blind* is still firmly plastered on more than a million men, women, and children in the United States, and according to the World Health Organization, 45 million worldwide. If you add in the people who have low vision that cannot be corrected, the number leaps to 10 million in the United States and 124 million around the world.

BLIND

When my research helped me peel off the label, I saw striking differences wherever I looked. As old Pilate says, I saw a rainbow.

There are first of all the countless personality traits that distinguish us one from another. Then there are the big life circumstances—gender, ethnic background, social class, religion or lack of it. There are talents, dreams, inclinations, the shape of the imagination. There are family members as well as the surrounding culture, whose assumptions and actions either liberate or imprison people who are blind. It matters greatly, for instance, whether a blind person lives in a Mexican village where parasite-borne blindness is common, in Paris during World War II when the French government leaned toward the fascist belief that only the able-bodied deserved employment, or, like my dad, in the United States in the thirties, forties, fifties, and sixties. Most people who write about their blindness take pains to claim their experiences only for themselves rather than generalizing. One example of many is the title of John Hull's memoir: *Touching the Rock: An Experience of Blindness.* Hull knows that his experience is only one of countless ways of being blind.

Each of these qualities or circumstances interacts differently with blindness, but to complicate the matter further, blindness is not just one condition. The American Foundation of the Blind lists on its website a whole alphabet of diseases, genetic conditions, environmental influences, and human mistakes that can cause blindness, each of them with its own pace, manifestations, and unique difficulties. The twilight zone between full sight and total blindness where my father lived for most of his life encompasses another range of conditions that block, narrow, or distort vision in often bizarre ways. (People with low vision describe looking at the world through one or two soda straws; seeing the world as an expressionist painting; being able to see one minute and not the next; looking out through lenses that seem to be smeared with

Vaseline.) People who are born blind or who go blind in early child-hood obviously experience their world and adapt to it differently from those who go blind gradually over many years or the rapidly growing number who are blinded by diseases that often strike in old age—glaucoma, macular degeneration, and diabetic retinopa-thy. It's important to look at these differences, if only to sort out the preventable from the nonpreventable causes of blindness. The World Health Organization says that three out of every four cases of blindness in developing countries are preventable or treatable and are closely linked with poverty, both as cause and effect.

I will examine several of these influential factors in other chapters. Here I want to consider the work men and women who are blind do—or, more often, don't get to do. The National Federation of the Blind reports the scandalous and terrifying fact that 70 percent of blind people of working age in the United States and more than 50 percent of the visually impaired are unemployed. Those of us lucky enough to have jobs we love that suit our talents and inclinations know how important work is to self-esteem and to our knowledge that we're helping to build the world. And even if we don't like our jobs, we gain confidence and even exhilaration from supporting ourselves, our families, and our communities. It's not accidental that we often ask each other, "What do you do for a *living*?" Among blind men and women, some want or need to live on Social Security or General Assistance. But five to seven out of every ten? Impossible. Like people with sight, people without sight are hungry for satisfying, creative, needed work that pays them a living wage and grants them autonomy.

My dad was never part of that grim unemployment statistic. He worked daily from boyhood until he died at age seventy. But men like him and work like his rarely appear in the stories and memoirs I've read, in historical accounts of notable blind people,

BLIND

or in recent media portrayals. This silence is unfortunate. Ordinary working-class people make up the vast majority of the blind population around the world, yet they rarely find themselves reflected in the mirrors of story and image.

Most people who write about blindness are obviously writers, men and women whose gift is scholarship, reading, the study and creation of languages and literature. There are the famous ones—Homer, Milton, James Joyce, James Thurber, Aldous Huxley, and John Howard Griffin, author of *Black Like Me*—and many who are less famous but who also live by their pens or computer keyboards and who have written books about their blindness—journalist Sally Wagner, poet Eleanor Clark, historian Robert Hine, *Time* magazine editor-in-chief Henry Grunwald, religious writer John Hull, philosopher and writer for the French Resistance Jacques Lusseyran. It might seem at first that ordinary men like my father have less to lose to blindness than do the many great literary people who were blind, or nearly so, for part or most of their lives. In his essay "Blindness," the Argentinean writer Jorge Luis Borges repeats like a refrain, "Blindness has not been for me a total misfortune; it should not be seen in a pathetic way," and even, "Blindness is a gift." He makes this bold assertion not only about himself but also about those other brave writers who "overcome blindness" to do their work. Milton had readers and his long-suffering daughters to take dictation; some writers used Braille or Braille typewriters; writers now have tapes, Dictaphones, talking books, high-tech magnifiers, and voice-sensitive computers. Nowhere in Borges' essay is there a blind farmer, grocery store owner, truck driver, highway builder, construction worker—all the people whose work must speak for them.

When I turn from Borges' elegant essay to my dad's halting letters to my mom (*his* refrain—"I don't know how to put things into words"), I find that the many kinds of work he did required sight in a way that literary work doesn't. My dad was a physical man, strong and agile. In his letters he describes the fun of pitching horseshoes with the guys on a rare free Sunday, and music with a good beat always set his feet to dancing. He could hoist a hundred-pound bag of potatoes or a bushel of carrots to his shoulder and walk lightly over our uneven yard from the garden to the market, one hand on his hip, the other balancing the load. During the three or four years before he got married, the years recorded in his letters, he describes hauling all over Minnesota and North Dakota anything that could be loaded in the box of his truck: coal, hay, grain, fence posts, vegetables, machinery, extra chairs to a movie theater where a prize fight film was being shown. Those years, his truck and his ability to drive and maintain it were essential to his livelihood. Eleven months after he and Mom got married, Judy, their first daughter, was born. When he was driving home from the hospital, the sun blinded him, and the police found him driving in the wrong lane, into the sparse morning traffic. They thought he was drunk, but the verdict was much worse: he couldn't see well enough to drive, even in rural North Dakota. When he lost his license, my dad lost his mobility and had to face one more dependency on his loving, willing wife as she got behind the wheel. A man who had hitchhiked, ridden freights, and driven across the top half of the United States and part of Canada and who carried in his mind memories of the Rockies and the Cascades must've felt himself doomed to the flatness of life in central North Dakota, "this godforsaken place." More dire still, he had lost an important way of supporting a family that now included a baby.

Borges writes that after he became almost blind he learned Anglo Saxon, Scandinavian, and Icelandic, and he marvels that Milton could compose and hold in his memory forty or fifty hendecasyllables of *Paradise Lost*, until a chance visitor stopped by who could write them down. My dad had a prodigious memory, too, and a love of the ring and swing of language. To his dying day, he could recite the poems he'd memorized in grade school. We grew up hearing him declaim "Barbara Fritchie"—" 'Shoot if you must this old gray head/But spare your country's flag,' she said"—and singing the dozens of songs he knew by heart and passed on to us. But poems and songs would not earn a living in Mandan, North Dakota. To greet the people who came to his grocery store/vegetable market, he had to memorize hundreds of names and voices; light, heavy, and halting footsteps; the names of seeds and vegetables—Early Ohio, Danvers Half Long, Straight Eight; the ring of a perfect watermelon; the price of every item in our store—Vienna sausages, antifreeze, used air compressors, that day's slightly over-the-hill bananas. He knew his carpenters' tools by touch, heft, sharpness, and position in his tool box. But this was all fleeting information that no daughter or visitor wrote down for him. In "Requa," her little-known short story about men scrabbling to get by during the Great Depression, Tillie Olsen finds poetry in tools and in the rhythms of manual labor:

> accurately threaded, reamed and chamfered   Shim Imperial flared
> cutters benders grinders beaders
> shapers notchers splicers reamers
> how many shapes and sizes
> how various, how cunning in application
> sharpening hauling sorting splicing
> burring chipping grinding cutting
> grooving drilling caulking sawing

But her insight into the poetry of manual labor is rare; and though my father loved fresh vegetables, his tools, and the work they could do, it wouldn't have occurred to him to shape their names into a poem. Even if he had, there are no anthologies to collect this concrete poetry and no Nobel Prizes to honor it.

In a ringing speech delivered in 1973 to the National Federation of the Blind, Dr. Kenneth Jernigan, then the Federation's president, challenged the perception among blind and sighted people alike that "the blind have moved through time and the world not only sightless but faceless, a people without distinguishing features, anonymous and insignificant, not so much as rippling the stream of history." This view is, he says, "not fact but fable, not truth but a lie." To counter this fabulous lie Jernigan describes the dazzling accomplishments of military strategists, road builders, scientists, mathematicians, lawyers, zoologists, theologians, all of them brilliant and productive. I didn't find my dad in that brilliant company. I found him in a few throw-away sentences near the end of Jernigan's speech:

> Isn't it true that most blind people throughout history have lived humdrum lives, achieving neither fame nor glory, and soon forgotten? Yes, it is true but for the sighted as well as for the blind. For the overwhelming majority of mankind (blind and sighted alike) life has been squalor and hard knocks and anonymity from as far back as anybody knows. There were doubtless blind peasants, blind housewives, blind shoemakers, blind businessmen, blind thieves, blind prostitutes, and blind holy men who performed as competently or as incompetently (and are now as forgotten) as their sighted contemporaries.

I'm not willing to settle for anonymity and forgetting.

I don't know my father, in part, because no one has told the story of people like him—ordinary people with disabilities who are amazing only in their fidelity, their refusal to give up, and the love for their families that kept them at hard, awkward, often unrewarding work all their lives. I didn't even find him in Frances Koestler's aptly titled book, *The Unseen Minority: A Social History of Blindness in the United States.* In this comprehensive, fact-laden study, Koestler traces the progress blind people have made from ancient times to the 1970s. But my dad appears only buried in statistics. He's among the people who *didn't* use a cane, have a guide dog, take mobility training or rehab, work in a sheltered workshop, or receive disability payments. In this fat book that tracks positive developments for blind men and women, he is a negative presence.

Now, in the twenty-first century, his life and the lives of many people with disabilities are again overshadowed and rendered invisible, this time by the stories of "supercrips" in history, literature, and the media. This is a name coined by other people with disabilities, and it contains a mixture of affection, humor, and envy for the supercrips themselves and derision for the awe and adulation that greet their supposedly heroic feats. Among the blind and visually impaired, they are musicians like Ray Charles and Stevie Wonder. They are athletes like twenty-year-old Rachel Scdoris, a legally blind musher who competed in the 2005 Iditarod, a thousand-mile sled-dog race from Anchorage to Nome, and Eric Weihenmayer, who has climbed most of the high mountains of the world, prefers climbing on ice, leads climbing expeditions, and on May 25, 2001, reached the summit of Mount Everest. (His climbing buddies call him "Super Blind Guy.") They are scholars like Tim Cordes, who graduated in 2005 in the top sixth of his class at the University of Wisconsin-Madison Medical School. He has his MD and now plans to get a PhD in biochemistry and might eventually become a psychiatrist. Along the way he earned a black belt in judo and Tae Kwan Do and learned to water ski and compose music. Blind supercrips have made their way into television ads whose makers are eager to show how inclusive they are in their sympathies. In a recent ad, a beautiful young woman kickboxes her opponent into submission then flips open her white cane and strides toward the people on the other side of the television screen, all of them amazed, wide-eyed, sighted. Since no blind person can see her leaps, her frighteningly accurate hands and feet, and her confident stride, the message is obviously for sighted people. What is that message? Maybe it's a warning to potential muggers: don't mess with a woman carrying a white cane unless you want your nose flattened by a well-aimed kick. If a blind woman can do this, think of what you, with your two eyes, can do. Or, perhaps, blind women can be champion kick boxers. Wonderful as they are, these people perform feats of artistry, athleticism, and scholarship that 99.9 percent of the population, sighted or blind, cannot match. Yet corporations and foundations are eager to back extraordinary athletes like Weihenmayer; his climbing gear sported Allegra and Power Bar labels, and the National Federation of the Blind supported the climb to the tune of a quarter of a million dollars. More than twenty corporate sponsors paid for his 2004 climbing expedition, in which he led six blind Tibetan teenagers up a twenty-three-thousand-foot mountain.

Supercrips themselves are the first to disclaim the adulation they receive and the idea that they and their accomplishments are heroic. When Eric Weihenmayer's young Tibetan climbers had to stop a thousand feet short of the summit of Lhakpa Ri, he was quick to assure them and the world tracking them on the Internet that the important accomplishment is not a mountain peak but their refusal to be limited by other people's ideas of what they can do. It's natural to be entranced and challenged by people who go beyond agreed-upon limits. Still, I fear that the hype over supercrips, rather than opening a wider space for other people with similar disabilities, only makes life harder for them. As Kathi Wolfe, a blind freelance writer, says, "If we hear enough such stories, we may feel defeated by the comparison. And trying to live up to the image can be just as damaging." As she says, "[when] one of us bursts into the cultural radar screen as a super-hero . . . all of us are expected to perform amazing feats." The day after Weihenmayer raised his arms high above Everest's icy summit, a friend asked Wolfe, with misplaced admiration, "So . . . when are you going to climb Mount Everest?" Like almost all of us, Wolfe sensibly answered, "*Never!*"

Crowds of blind people will not become musical prodigies, for contrary to the mythology surrounding blindness, it doesn't automatically confer perfect pitch or musical talent. Nor will they flock to medical school or PhD programs in biochemistry. Still fewer will head north to Alaska next March. Besides Rachel Scdoris, only seventy-eight mushers competed in 2005, and more people have reached the summit of Mount Everest than have crossed the finish line of the Iditarod.

The media glare surrounding supercrips can easily blind all of us to the modest accomplishments of a man like my father. When I set him alongside blind mountain climbers, physicians, legendary musicians and performers, writers, and resistance fighters, I'm tempted to think that he wasn't as brave as they were, wasn't as stubborn, faith filled, flexible, imaginative, or talented. For these are the qualities people who "overcome blindness" appear to have. But in my memory of him, he had all these qualities. I can't remember a single time when he showed the opposite traits. Though he was far from being a perfect husband and father, he wasn't a coward or a quitter, faithless, rigid, dull, or stupid.

Why then does he appear in my memory as a defeated man whose self-confidence ebbed almost to nothing by the time I left home? I think it has something to do with the time in which he lived his life. There were no Special Olympics, no Americans with Disabilities Act, certainly no corporate sponsors eager to bankroll a man who in his earlier, sighted years had climbed Mount Rainier but who was now only trying to support his family. In a black and white picture I have of him, he's standing in front of our grocery store. It must be Sunday morning because he's wearing his white shirt and good pants and shoes rather than the blue chambray workshirt, Oshkosh bib overalls, and heavy work shoes he wore the other six days of the week. His gray-white hair is blowing, and his forehead is white down to his bushy eyebrows. The rest of his face and his hands are very dark. He always wore an Irish workingman's cap, flat, with a visor to shield his eyes from the sun's glare. (RP, until it makes you blind, makes your eyes painfully sensitive to bright lights; the sun or oncoming headlights blind you.) His big, strong hands are holding each other, and his eyes, behind his futile glasses, are looking intently to where my mother stands with the box Kodak. He isn't smiling. Behind him, reflected in the store window, are several of his children. Nailed to the door of our market is the only endorsement he ever got: a tin sign advertising regular and king-size Chesterfields.

During my dad's lifetime, there were few supercrips. Instead, he faced pity and suffocatingly low expectations on the part of educators, psychologists, and social theorists. In *Hope Deferred: Public Welfare and the Blind,* Jacobus tenBroek and Floyd Matson describe the prevailing attitudes toward employment for the blind in the forties and fifties. They quote educators, historians, and psychologists who assert that blindness is most often accompanied by passivity and a desire to be taken care of. Thomas Cutsforth, a psychologist specializing in blindness, wrote in 1950: "The blind, like other frustrated personalities, trade the birthright of self-assurance that goes with aggressive action, the courage that goes with anger, and the audacity that goes with rage for ineffectual action, compliant passivity, and the self-contempt of a dependent." Schools for the blind seem to have based their philosophy, curriculum, and methods on this distorted perception. *From Homer to Helen Keller: A Social and Educational Study of the Blind* by Richard French is a 1932 text many considered a classic. French makes the mouth-filling pronouncement that "there is little in an industrial way that a blind person can do at all that cannot be done better and more expeditiously by people with sight." He grants that a few blind people are skilled at "basketry, weaving, knitting, broom- and brush-making, and chair-caning"; but even in these crafts they can't possibly compete with sighted people. With his tongue in his cheek, French calls piano tuning and massage "higher" callings, for which the blind need special accommodations. But "the learned professions, including teaching," are out of reach for all but the most talented, the bravest, those determined "to win at all costs."

These well-meaning experts, who claim that their conclusions rest on long years of experience with blind students, workers, and patients, assert that it's cruel and hypocritical to hold out to most people who are blind the unreasonable hope that they can be productive workers "in the sighted world." Only the superblind dare to venture beyond those stifling limits. Cutsforth scolds anyone who tries to persuade the sighted world that the blind "are normal individuals without vision." With what has to be unconscious irony, he says, "This desperate whistling in the dark does more damage than good." These learned opinions worked their way into everyday life, reinforcing ancient prejudices, so that blind people met pity, condescension, and frequent rebuffs. TenBroek and Matson document a few that happened in 1957: for no reason except her or his blindness, a blind person couldn't rent a room at the

YMCA, donate blood, be a district judge, rent a safety-deposit box, perform jury duty, practice teach, buy a plane ticket, serve as student body president, or hold a job he had already done capably for several years.

My dad certainly never read these descriptions of himself and his capabilities, but he met similar preconceptions in the people who came to our store and in us, his family. Still, until he lost his front tooth, he always whistled in the dark, and his independence, audacity, anger, and competitiveness challenged anyone who told him what he could or couldn't do. Besides my dad, we knew three blind people: Darrel and Mildred Kline, who lived a mile down the road from us, and Lloyd Robertson, who occasionally took on the thankless task of tuning our old piano. All three of them had gone to the school for the blind in Bathgate, North Dakota, where they had learned to read and write Braille, use white canes, and support themselves. Lloyd was, as I said, a piano tuner; Darrel caned chairs, wove beautiful, sturdy rag rugs, and ran a trailer court. All of them were happier than my dad because they were more reconciled to their blindness. Darrel often urged Dad to go to Camp Grassick, a week-long summer camp run by the North Dakota Association of the Blind, to get mobility and job training. He always refused. I can guess at some of his reasons. Acknowledging his blindness would mean giving up hope that doctors would find a cure for RP, a mirage always beckoning and always receding in the distance. It would betray his remaining sight. Almost blinded by macular degeneration late in life, *Time* editor Henry Grunwald didn't try to learn Braille because, as he writes, "It implies total blindness and would mean a denial of the sight I still have." For Grunwald and my dad, it would mean being a quitter.

My dad, a gambling man, bet on underdogs. I can still hear his glad shout when Rocky Marciano knocked out Jersey Joe Walcott in the thirteenth round to become the heavyweight champion of the world. The smart money in Mandan was on Walcott. Dad's five dollars were riding on Marciano. All his life, he bet on himself to beat the odds. Most people in the thirties, forties, and fifties didn't think much about vocation, dream jobs, or self-fulfillment. During the Great Depression and after, men and women were glad to have any job that kept them off welfare. I never asked either of my parents what job they would have chosen if they could have done anything they wanted. I don't know if Dad wanted to be a farmer, a trucker, a market gardener, a general store operator, a fireworks salesman. But I know he didn't want the jobs or the dependence he expected the school for the blind to offer him.

Since my dad put up his lonely fight, working conditions and possibilities have changed enormously for men and women who are blind. The best evidence of these changes is that the philosophies and practices I just described now sound as if they came out of the Dark Ages, as they surely did. Today, individual blind men and women are succeeding in almost every occupation you can name, including the most improbable. For example, in 2005 the University of California-Berkeley Art Museum presented an exhibition of the works of several blind and visually impaired photographers, sculptors, and multimedia artists, whose works challenge the current wisdom about sight and the act of seeing and redefine the role and architecture of an art museum. Helped by innovative training programs, wonderful new technologies, and the legal muscle of the Americans with Disabilities Act, signed into law in 1990, blind people are becoming teachers, architects, physicians, lawyers, and coaches. A trickle of stories has begun to appear about ordinary people doing ordinary jobs: physical therapy, running a sporting goods store, farming, car repair, carpentry. In 1995 a crew of blind computer engineers led by Ted Henter devised the screen-reading program JAWS for Windows that translates not just text but icons and graphics into speech. Instead of a mouse, operators use key strokes directed by the computer's voice. This innovation, which has been translated into ten world languages and has twenty-five-thousand users, opened up thousands of Windows-dependent jobs to blind people. In fact, JAWS stands for Job Accessibility with Speech. The Internet, enhanced by voice-activated software, lets blind people around the world talk to each other, offering encouragement and practical hints. (How do you deal with the class troublemaker, the kid cheating on a test, the stacks of essays, the nervous parents? What kind of camera do you use, and how do you develop your prints?) As Erik Weihenmeyer says, "There is a blurry line separating what the world sees as impossible" and those things "we know in our hearts to be possible." He adds that when he "strove to look beyond convention," he realized that there isn't just one way to climb a mountain of ice—the sighted way. And if there are many ways to climb a mountain, there must also be an infinite number of ways to do the more mundane jobs most blind people aspire to.

Blind mountain climbers, champion skiers, MDs, and police detectives all make imaginable what had been unimaginable a few years ago, make thinkable what had been unthinkable. Because Eric Weihenmayer climbed high mountains, six blind kids thought they might be able to do it too. And this was in Tibet, where, until 1998 when Sabriye Tenberken and Paul Kronenberg opened their school, Braille without Borders, blind Tibetan children were considered sinful or demonic, and shamed parents often hid them away in dark rooms. Thanks to many people who refuse to hide, blind people are becoming more visible to the sighted world and, therefore, less strange and frightening. New organizations abound to take blind people skiing, rock climbing, and kayaking and to put the latest technology under their fingertips. But no one can ski forever, and if blind people can't find meaningful work, none of these helpful and imaginative developments will make their lives whole.

It's important to take another look at that stubborn 50–70 percent unemployment rate. Virtually every memoir or autobiography I've read, even the most recent, records struggles to get and keep jobs, in spite of education and specialized training in mobility and independence, adequate skills, and high motivation, sometimes even in spite of brilliance. With humor, anger, and great honesty, these writers tell of losing jobs for flimsy reasons, even with the protection of the ADA. Of course, mountain climbers were certain that Erik Weihenmayer would never make it to the top of Everest. One climber from another team wanted the distinction of taking "the first picture of the dead blind guy." Given the 90 percent failure rate of Everest climbers, his skepticism is understandable, even if his crassness isn't. It's more disheartening to learn that Erik applied for dozens of low-skilled jobs to help pay his way through Harvard. He never landed one, not even as a dishwasher, though he was frequently lectured on the wisdom of accepting his limitations. He says of this often repeated experience: "I did choke down an important lesson, that people's perceptions of our limitations are more damaging than those limitations themselves, and it was the hardest lesson I ever had to swallow."

Deborah Wingwall, one of the photographers in the Berkeley exhibit, says that most people look admiringly at her photographs and ask, "How do you do that?" but they really mean, "You can't do that." New MD Tim Cordes was turned down by several of the medical schools he applied to, in spite of graduating from Notre Dame as valedictorian with a 3.99 GPA in biochemistry; he had also garnered a couple of years' experience in biomedical research and recommenders who raved about his abilities and motivation.

Most distressing of all, some counselors and psychologists still advocate dependency. In the 1997 documentary *In the Mind of the Beholder,* Peter Damien, a recently blinded man in his thirties or early forties, says that a counselor urged him to go on Social Security Disability, retire, and "sit around and get a tan and go to Palm Springs all the time." Wanting to keep his self-esteem intact, he refused. It could be that the counselor hated his job and couldn't wait to retire and start working on his tan; he might even have thought privately that the silver lining in the cloud of blindness is that you can retire early or, better yet, don't have to work at all. But what a narrow, distorted view of blindness and work that is!

Many blind people are trying to shatter the stereotypes surrounding them and two opposite but equally destructive attitudes: pity that ignores or diminishes their real gifts and a false belief that anything is possible for them if they just try as hard as and are as brave as Helen Keller, Eric Weihenmayer, and the other superscrips. In fact, Marc Mauer, the president of the National Federation of the Blind, has proposed that Eric replace Helen Keller as "a contemporary symbol for blindness." The latter attitude ignores real gifts, accomplishments, and possibilities as surely as a demeaning pity that relegates all blind people to the "suitable labor" of caning chairs or selling pencils, or worse yet, permanent disability checks and empty, useless hands.

In central Minnesota where I live, the last receding glacier left behind sandy soil thickly seeded with rocks. Every year the winter freeze and snow and the spring thaw turn up a crop of stones, even in fields that were picked clean the previous spring. On the farms around here, kids used to stay out of school to pick rocks before their parents could plant corn or soybeans. The stereotypes and myths, the awkwardness and rigidity I find in myself and in some workplaces are like those rocks, turned up year after year by the thaw that has warmed the lives of blind people in many other ways. Stephen Kuusisto, author of the brilliant memoir, *The Planet of the Blind,* might call these rocks "the sighted world's patterned responses to blindness." I want to pick them up, turn them over in my hands, feel their shape and heft, and think of ways they can be cleared away so real growth can happen, not only for blind men and women but even more for the sighted people they work with and for.

During the women's movement of the 1970s and 1980s I often read some version of this statement on bumper stickers and posters: "In order to be considered as good as a man at your job, you have to be twice as good. Fortunately, this is not difficult." While I appreciate the statement's defiant humor, I know it's not true for most women. Nor is it true for members of any marginalized group trying to win equal access to training, jobs, and professions, and, once they land the job, equal treatment, salary, and opportunities for advancement. Certainly, to get and hold a job, women and members of ethnic minorities must be fully qualified and motivated. But they shouldn't have to be twice as good as the average worker. It's true that most of us don't use all our intelligence, skill, grace, and charm; it would do us and the world good if we were to reach higher and dig deeper. But it's also true that all of us have limitations that won't budge, which brings me back to blind workers and supercrips. We dare not say out loud that we expect blind people, like other people with disabilities, to prove their value in the workplace by being better in every way than the average worker: more skillful or intelligent, more tenacious, nicer, braver. In *How Do You Kiss a Blind Girl?*, Sally Wagner tells how her well-meaning friends tried to cheer her on by invoking brave blind people. "There must have been thousands of them," she says, "because everybody knew at least one." She adds, "It's tough to adjust well when you're surrounded by nothing but the bravest of role models. Sometimes I'd have given my eye teeth to hear about just one lily-livered chicken like me." Besides the distinctive array of limitations every person must make peace with, women and men who are blind must also accept the genuine limitations blindness creates. It puts some jobs out of reach entirely—pro baseball player, motorcycle cop, over-the-road trucker, airplane pilot—and requires accommodations for many other jobs. Blind workers must often find human helpers and adaptive techniques and technologies and persuade coworkers and supervisors to modify the office, classroom, or factory and even the job itself to help the worker do a good job (though not necessarily a super job). This negotiation demands a hefty store of initiative and self-confidence on the workers' part and an equally good dose of imagination and adaptability on the part of sighted bosses and colleagues. But several attitudes, all of them buried just underground, get in the way of the hopeful situation I've just outlined.

Some of us begrudge others the accommodations we didn't get. It's trendy now to claim that everyone is disabled in some way and to lump all handicaps together. It follows that if anyone gets a break, everyone should. Richard Bolles, in his widely used career-counseling series, *What Color Is Your Parachute?* reinforces this trend. From 1970 to 1991 his book included a useful section on job-hunting tips for people with disabilities. He has since relegated this information to a pamphlet that must be ordered separately and that many libraries and career counseling centers don't have. In the 2000 edition of *What Color,* he devotes two pages to handicaps. Blindness appears in his capacious list, right up there with being too beautiful, too thin, too educated, or an excon. Needless to say, his generic advice is useless to employers and job hunters alike. What I'm saying is not special pleading on behalf of blind people. It could apply just as easily to a range of other real physical or mental handicaps.

The presence of a blind person at the next desk or work table can pull fears to the surface. He or she is a reminder that each of us is one disease or one accident away from blindness. In fact, the World Health Organization warns of "a rising tide of blindness" as the population of developing countries ages. We see in our blind colleague our possible future self, a damaged self we'd rather not contemplate.

We may also fear that our resilient prejudices will reveal themselves in our words and actions; we won't know what to do or say that won't offend. We'll blunder many times a day, offering too much help or none at all, being too critical or too complimentary, laughing too much or being afraid to laugh at all, talking too loudly or whispering, talking about but not to. We might even fall prey to the old notion that blindness brings with it a lack of intelligence or awareness and that most jobs—certainly *my* job—are impossible for a blind person to do, even with all the adaptations in the world. I might praise my blind coworker lavishly for small accomplishments but assume that the blind as a group are automatically barred even from jobs they have been doing quietly and capably for decades. For instance, until 1997 blind people couldn't be certified to teach other blind people to travel with white canes, and then only with a sighted assistant. This restriction was in place in spite of the fact that they'd been doing it for years, using nonvisual methods that the certifying organization didn't recognize.

I may discover in myself the opposite notion, that intuition automatically replaces eyesight, enabling a blind person's finely tuned sixth sense to turn me inside out. This is another old stereotype picked up and made graphic by the short-lived 2005 television series *Blind Justice*. Jim Dunbar is a New York police detective blinded in the line of duty. A year later, he returns to the NYPD and asks to be reinstated. The police chief and his fellow detectives are skeptical at first, testing his skills, his manhood, and his ability to avoid the obstacles they put in his path. But in true TV form, Detective Dunbar proves himself week after week. He has an expressive guide dog named Hank with whom he travels all over New York, but most of the time when he's investigating a crime, he holds his partner's arm and asks her to describe the scene to him. He carries a gun. Except for the gun this series takes pains to present somewhat realistic and interesting information and to introduce new technology (such as a hand-held currency reader), but it also lapses into stereotypes of the supercrip variety. For instance, Dunbar sometimes solves crimes because of his heightened sense of smell or hearing or, worse yet, because of a sixth sense signaled by a flash of white light.

We might be afraid a blind colleague will slow us down, when most jobs depend on ever-increasing speed, and that we'll respond with irritation and impatience. We might be like Stephen Kuusisto's English teacher at the University of Iowa who tells Kuusisto that he doesn't belong in the college or in this teacher's graduate class because he needs extra time to do the reading. To which Kuusisto says, "Of course, you're right. And I suppose Milton, Homer, James Joyce, they couldn't have taken a course in this department either?" Only by getting the college's dean to enforce the ADA does he get to finish the course.

While these grudges and fears are common, the memoirs I've read convince me that they are neither inevitable nor changeless. Stephen Kuusisto writes appreciatively about his teachers at Guiding Eye for the Blind, a school in Yorktown Heights, New York, that matches up guide dogs and blind people and teaches them to work as a team. There for the first time he met sighted teachers who, as he says, "respect blindness." Unlike his obtuse English professor, these teachers "work you hard while you're in residence, and they admire your breakthrough" but without "an ounce of the patronizing or the sentimental." If these sighted teachers can learn, so can I, but not if I ponder blindness only in the sanctuary of my mind. As with all people, we learn to distinguish what hurts from what helps in the rub of everyday exchanges. Unless I truly want the blind, those undifferentiated millions, to be blind, that is, *out of sight, out of the way, secret, obscure,* I must learn. That can happen only if my college, for example, is willing to hire blind English, math, zoology, photography, or music teachers and then make needed accommodations, person by person.

In a chapter of *The Unseen Minority* called "Mobility, Key to Independence," Koestler writes that in the forties and fifties most blind people depended "on human guides to navigate safely." This choice came, she says, from "the self-denigrating belief that blindness should be made as inconspicuous as possible, and that the use of a dog guide or a distinctive cane attracted undesirable public attention." Many people have written eloquently about the freedom canes and dogs give them—freedom to move about the city and the world and, most of all, the freedom to stop pretending they can see. Thousands more are freely and openly blind, canes and dogs boldly accompanying them to and from work. Eric Weihenmayer for one succeeded on many fronts when he stopped pretending he had sight and began "to build systems that allowed him to excel without it." He considers it tragic that some blind people still try to "pass." "What's the point of that?" he asks.

I've often wished that my dad had listened to Darrel Kline and gone to Camp Grassick. Being in the company of honest, funny blind men and women might have eased his loneliness, muffled round with silence. He might even have learned to laugh in the teeth of blindness. I wish he had learned to use a cane and the adaptive devices that were available in his lifetime. I wish he could have said, "I'm blind," without hating the words and maybe himself. Most of all, I wish he could have been happy instead of always being braced for trouble, a battered, bare-knuckle fighter with his dukes up, ready to take on all comers. He taught his children one way to be blind, but I don't think it's a confident, free, open way. I wish he could have helped change the myths and metaphors attracted by the gravitational pull of blindness instead of simply resisting them. But for reasons I've been suggesting all along, he couldn't. Again, I find that in his loneliness he's not alone.

For understandable and practical reasons people from North Dakota to Tibet did and still do hide their canes and hang on to a friendly arm, though I hesitate to attribute that choice to self-denigration, as Frances Koestler does. For example, Ginger Lee, a sixth-grade teacher in Oshkosh, Wisconsin, says, "I know I'm successful when people don't know I'm blind." Blind artists such as Deborah Wingwall want the simple justice of hearing their work assessed on its merits and themselves defined by their work rather than by their disability. They don't want the patronizing praise often lavished on blind people for doing what everyone else in the workplace is doing: Good work for a blind artist/teacher/ computer programmer/financial analyst/grocer! Nor do they want to be included in a litany of exceptions, or, to borrow Tillie Olsen's word, *Only's*.

Blind workers have another reason for caution. They are well aware of the fears and resentments, the rock-hard patterned responses, their blindness can trigger. My sister Coreen, a gifted fourth-grade teacher, rarely tells the parents of her students that she's visually impaired because she's afraid some of them will assume that she is inept and ineffective. She knows she might be wrong about them, but she needs and wants both the job and the trust of the parents; she can't risk honesty. So, it seems safer to pass, to prove herself as a competent and reliable worker, and then some day say causally, "Oh, by the way, I'm legally blind."

But the greatest fear for a person with a highly visible cane or a big, kind dog is never getting a job at all. If someone had asked me when I began this book whether a blind man or woman could do my job—teaching literature and writing to undergrads at a liberal arts college—I would have said a regretful but definite no, suggesting instead jobs like wine taster or perfume sniffer. Now, with no reservations except for the stringent professional ones I apply to any candidate for my job, I'd say an unqualified yes. In fact, Stephen Kuusisto became an assistant professor of English at the Ohio State University at Columbus, teaching the same creative writing classes I've taught, plus innovative literature courses, such as the Disability Experience in the Contemporary World and the Disability Memoir: Autobiography, Politics, and Personal Identity. But this job came after years of searching. Until he was thirty-nine, Kuusisto lived recklessly in the twilight between blindness and sight, always pretending to be able to see much more than he really could. Then he learned to use a cane and shortly after got Corky, his guide dog. As he says, "At the age of thirty-nine I learn to walk upright." But when he returned to his hometown, he and Corky pounded the streets for over a year, meeting pessimism about employment around every corner, both in himself and in the social workers who tried to help him find a job. He lived on Social Security and food stamps, or as he calls it, "state-sponsored hope." Over a lifetime, an unemployed blind person costs U.S. society almost $1 million in SSDI and lost taxes. That loss is trivial next to the loss of the intelligence, manual skill, tenacity, and inventiveness blind people can bring to their jobs. Worst of all, if the blind are unable to give their gifts, the gifts turn to stone in their hands. When Kuusisto was looking for work, he wondered if he would ever "discover the joyous striving that necessarily defines a strong and good life." If anyone needs a reason to open work places wide to the blind, those words should provide it, for that's what most of us want for ourselves and for those we respect and love.

FOUR

Turn a Blind Eye

To deliberately ignore something when you know
it is going on

GUIDED BY MY DAD, my family was proudly Irish in a
North Dakota community made up almost entirely
of German Russians and Bohemians. We didn't
parade our Irishness only on St. Patrick's Day. We were Irish
year round and certain that this was the best nationality, with
my mother's German heritage coming in a distant second. We
called ourselves Irish Germans rather than Americans and were
pleased to tell our classmates that our Grandpa Faulkner came
from Dublin. Irish pride was incarnated in our dad. We heard
it in the remnants of a brogue and words no one else used: "Ye
blackguards!" "I dasn't!" "Holy jumping balls!", an exclamation
we repeated without knowing what it meant because we loved
its jauntiness and the happiness and humor in our dad's voice
when he said it. He sang happy-sad songs about going back
to old Ireland as he step danced around the kitchen: "I'll Take

You Home Again, Kathleen" and "It's a Long Way to Tipperary."
At his wake we sang "Galway Bay," that Irish American song of
longing for the green island he had never seen, its trout streams
and turf fires, its defiant spirit. For Dad, if Ireland and Heaven
weren't identical, they were at least close neighbors. He loved the
Friday night prize fights from Madison Square Garden and told us
tales of the great Irish boxers of the past: John L. Sullivan, Gentle-
man Jim Corbett, Jack Dempsey, Gene Tunney. Stories about his
early life were filled with the names of his Irish neighbors—Kelly,
McManus, Maloney, Murphy, Shea—all of them apparently high
spirited, fun loving, and ready for devilment or a fight. The dark
side of this Irish pride was an implacable hatred of the English
that didn't seem to require explanation or justification.

There was another dark side, though as a child I didn't see it
for what it was. Dennis Faulkner had a complicated and contradictory attitude toward authority of all kinds, both his own and that
which social norms, the Catholic Church, and the government
exerted over him, or tried to. He was both an engaged citizen and
a law breaker. My mother and all of us kids had to learn to walk
through this tangle of contradictions without stumbling. It wasn't
easy, for Dad's actions often demanded that we turn a blind eye
to his reckless, sometimes callous, disregard for the law and for the
consequences of his actions.

Dad believed in democracy and in the importance of each person's
involvement in the political process. He was always interested in
politics and as well informed as he could be from listening to news
broadcasts and talking to the people who came in our store. As a
young man he had organized farmers for the Nonpartisan League,
a movement that began in 1915 in North Dakota to unite farmers
against the exploitation and price manipulation happening at every
point from field to market, in grain elevators, flour mills, packing

houses, stockyards, and the cold storage industry. He quit when it seemed to him that the League was anti-Catholic. As a staunch New Deal Democrat, he expected the government to help create economic justice. In North Dakota, which has been predominantly Republican since the 1940s, my dad always voted a straight Democratic ticket because, as he said, the Democrats were for the little guy. Voting wasn't easy for my mom and dad. Because we lived outside the Mandan city limits, we had to drive twenty miles to a country schoolhouse where my mother read the ballot to my dad, office by office, measure by measure. There was no chance that their votes would win the election for the Democrats, but it never occurred to either of them to stay home on election day. He was fiercely American, so, in the 1950s, when the charismatic Bishop Fulton J. Sheen and Senator Joe McCarthy—good Irishmen, both of them—led the attack on atheistic Communism, my dad hung on their words.

Dad apparently believed in the rule of law. He expected honesty and obedience from his children and patriotism and integrity from elected officials. Why, then, was our grocery store/gas station/vegetable market a blind for a variety of illegal activities? From under the counter, my dad sold bootleg whiskey and cheap wine to several Mandan Indians, who would otherwise have resorted to lemon extract or antifreeze. Sometimes my dad's lawbreaking was playful, a game to see what he could get away with. My brother, Dennie, remembers the time a truck hauling gallon jugs of apple cider overturned in our driveway. Hundreds of cars and trucks whizzed by our house on Interstate Highway 10, a two-lane road without much of a shoulder. On that lucky day, the cider truck hit the gravel, skidded, and landed on its side in the ditch. Most of the jugs shattered, but there were a few dozen survivors, which the trucker offered to my dad for next to nothing. Always alert for something he could sell at a nice profit, he bought the cider and stored it in our all-purpose cellar. It hadn't dawned on Dad that the accident might have broken the seals on the jugs until the cider started to ferment, brown foam oozing from under the caps and a pungent apple smell mixing with the familiar moldy smell of the cellar. Just as my dad was wondering how he'd unload fifty gallons of vinegar, he happened to taste the brew. It had transformed itself into delicious, potent hard cider. He could easily sell it to his Indian customers for a dollar a gallon. Mom's objections were futile. Dad probably considered the whole deal a stroke of good Irish luck: he could make a little money in a way that looked legal but wasn't.

These sales were doubly illegal because Dad didn't have a liquor license and, much worse in the North Dakota of the 1940s, Indians were forbidden by law to buy, sell, or consume alcohol. I didn't question my dad's explanation for the ban, which was also the explanation given by the lawmakers: Indians have wild blood, easily riled by booze. Dad offered no explanations at all for peddling illegal liquor or for selling dangerous firecrackers every Fourth of July, a defiance of the law that jeopardized our livelihood and our family.

Selling fireworks was and still is legal in North Dakota. Every June, my dad ordered huge stocks of Roman candles, sky rockets, and many varieties of exploding shells. In the long, beautiful North Dakota evenings, as soon as it got dark, he shot off a few demos. He couldn't see them, but the cars passing on Highway 10 could, and so could his kids. He wanted us to be able to accurately and dramatically describe each item to our customers. If I had to, I could still give a spiel about three-stage shells, phosphorescent parachutes, and exploding helicopters. But my dad didn't stop with the legal stuff. He also sold cherry bombs, bulldog salutes, and M80s—huge firecrackers that could blow off a man's hand or destroy a child's eye. He demonstrated those, too, and some evenings our yard sounded like a battleground as cherry bombs exploded under tin cans, shooting them far into the sky.

I don't know where the cops were on those June evenings. For all I know, they were among the customers. Obviously the word had got around town that Faulkner's was the place to buy illegal fireworks. I must have known that an informer is lower than the lowest criminal, so I lied, big-eyed and innocent, when young men asked me if my daddy sold "the big stuff." After all, they could have been undercover cops. Without understanding why our father broke the law, my mom, sisters, brother, and I covered for him.

But all of us were terrified of the explosives Dad hid in the attic and in the belly of the piano, an old, tone-deaf upright with a cracked sound board. We knew he was risking lawsuits, imprisonment, and the loss of our home. As Coreen once whispered to Mona, if they caught him, they'd even take the piano as an innocent accomplice to crime. One Fourth of July the sheriff came out from town claiming that a teenager had bought big firecrackers from my dad, lit one, stuck it down the barrel of a rifle, and lost his eye when he peered into the barrel to see why the firecracker hadn't exploded. Dad denied everything; and the minute the sheriff left, he got rid of the rest of his stash. But he couldn't ease our terror. In my nightmares, I saw his hands blown off and the stumps of his arms burning. I didn't let myself think about the kid with the ruined eye, who might or might not have bought his firecrackers at Faulkner's Market.

As a child, I simply lived with these contradictions and inconsistencies and tried not to get caught in them. In recent years, I've tried to understand my dad's reasons, which he never bothered to explain and may not have understood himself. Maybe bootleg liquor and illegal firecrackers were just another way to make a quick buck. Maybe he realized by age fifty that he'd never devise a way to get us out of our semi-poverty and decided that if he couldn't make a decent living legally, he was justified in making one illegally. Maybe he considered the law forbidding Indians to buy alcohol unjust. Maybe breaking the law, especially in flamboyant ways that other men secretly admired, was a blind man's way of asserting his manhood.

While all of these reasons probably came into play I realize now that all along I'd been focusing too narrowly. Of course I knew that Dad's blindness came to him from Ireland, but for most of my life, when I looked toward his and our Irish heritage, I saw it as a source of confidence, strength, and joy. I didn't see terror, oppression, famine, and a poverty of body, mind, and spirit that no songs or light-footed dances could ease. When I began to study the Great Famine that afflicted Ireland from 1845 to 1850 and its legacy, I saw psychological and social patterns that stunned me with their familiarity. I saw my father's attitudes and actions, especially regarding authority, writ large in the big world of the Irish Catholic people who immigrated to the United States during the Famine and in the following decades. I saw the same shocking contradictions and, finally, a devastating, deeply buried logic.

In spite of all the stories my father told us when we were growing up, I learned very little about his father, James Faulkner from Dublin, and nothing at all about the Great Famine, even though I know now that all four of my Irish great-grandparents lived through its devastation and survived to build homes and raise families. I went to Ireland hoping to fill in a few of the tantalizing gaps in our family story. I thought my grandfather's early life might provide some clues to my dad's contradictory personality and character. In fact, I thought my dad might have inherited his scofflaw tendencies from his father. Maybe James Faulkner was a Fenian—a radical republican on the run from the government—or at least a criminal with the peelers on his tail. I didn't find my grandfather's story in Ireland. What I did find was infinitely more revealing. I found the story of the Great Famine and began to understand that it was a crucial shaping force in my ancestors' lives, and through them—by their actions, their words, their silences—my father's life.

From old census records, obituaries, stray comments in *The History of Millerville* by Karl Klein, and a hand-written family tree, I've pieced together a rough version of the Kelly-Maloney-Faulkner story. There are, of course, numerous inconsistencies in dates and places, but I'm not as interested in the exact chronology of my ancestors' lives as in its familiar immigrant shape.

My great-grandfather Dennis Maloney was born in County Tipperary around 1831–1833. In 1855 he came to the United States, settling for a few years in Pittsfield in western Massachusetts. In 1867 he met and married Elizabeth Kelly, who had come to Pittsfield from County Monaghan with her mother and three brothers. Elizabeth was about twenty-two when they married, and Dennis at least ten years older. Within the next couple of years, they moved to Minneapolis, then known as St. Anthony, and had their first child, my grandmother Julia.

In 1868 or 1869 they bundled up their baby and headed northwest by ox cart to stake a claim in Leaf Valley Township, near Alexandria, Minnesota. Dennis and Elizabeth, or Bessie, were among the earliest settlers, claiming their 160 acres in what came to be called "Irish Corner." They were surrounded by the Shea, Murphy, Kelly, Lannigan, Mullins, Comerford, and McManus families, most of them straight from Ireland, and some from Dennis and Bessie's home counties. This tight group was in the minority in this mostly German and Norwegian section of the state. Dennis and Bessie had eight children, of whom six survived. Bessie's mother lived with them until she died at eighty-six, and so did their granddaughter, my Aunt Bessie, in that accepted nineteenth-century tradition of relatives taking a child or two when there are too many or the mother isn't well. Dennis Maloney was obviously a good farmer. In the 1870 Douglas County census, the value of his land and property is listed at four hundred dollars; in 1924, his son John took over the farm, listing its value at ten thousand dollars.

My grandfather James Faulkner, the oldest of ten children, was born in 1868 or 1869 in Rahana, County Louth, a townland in the beautiful hills and valleys northwest of Dublin. At some point, the family moved into a tenement in the port city of Kingstown (now Dun Laoghaire.) Somewhere between 1885 and 1888 young James worked his way across the Atlantic. His parents and siblings lived and died in Ireland, and James never saw them again. Somehow, he too landed in Leaf Valley Township, where he married Julia Maloney, who received eighty acres of land from her father. In their 1889 wedding picture, they're looking sternly at the camera. Julia is clutching Jim's arm; Jim is clutching his hat. Both are dressed in conventional nineteenth-century wedding finery. They too bore and raised eight children; my dad, Dennis, was number four, born in 1895.

This commonplace immigrant story would not bear telling except for one crucial fact: all but one of my great-grandparents were born shortly before or in the very year that the Great Hunger began to ravage Ireland. They and at least some part of their families lived through it and survived the terrible aftermath. County Monaghan and County Tipperary were among the areas that were especially hard hit, but no part of Ireland escaped starvation, disease, and eviction. The other Irish families who settled in Leaf Valley must have had similar histories—histories no one talked about. It's this eerie silence I'm trying to understand.

From my father's stories, I gather that the Irish clan that settled the southwest corner of Leaf Valley Township played, worked, and worshipped together. They had no Irish Catholic Church, so they went to the staunchly German Church of the Seven Dolors in Millerville. In his history, Karl Klein complains that unlike later Polish settlers, the Irish never bothered to learn German, even though they came to the Millerville church every week for sixty years and sat dutifully through German preaching. My dad's songs, dances, language, and friendships suggest that this clan resisted easy assimilation into Minnesota German culture.

My dad knew his grandparents well, and they lived relatively long lives. Dennis Maloney was around seventy-three when he died, and Bessie was eighty-seven. What's more, these were storytelling people. On the rare occasions that my aunts and uncle came to visit us in North Dakota, riotous stories from their childhoods filled our little house. Where, then, are the stories of the Famine, an event so catastrophic that it changed Ireland and its people forever? My ancestors must have brought personal memories and family stories with them when they sailed from Ireland. They seem to have passed on to their children and grandchildren pride, longing, an ancient hatred of the English, both a passion for justice and strangely twisted attitudes toward law and authority. But they didn't pass on the story, the history that would ease our bewilderment and help my generation understand a man like my father.

Drawn on by these questions and puzzling gaps, I've read dozens of accounts of the Famine years—1845–50—by Irish and Irish American historians, economists, political analysts, journalists, poets, and novelists. I read about the ideologies and resulting decisions that led inexorably to the Famine and the rationalizations that followed it. Among dozens of discoveries, two seem especially revealing as I try to understand my father. I discovered the burden of silence and the long roots of hatred.

Until very recently, silence about the Famine was pervasive. The story of the Great Hunger was buried not just by my family but by the whole generation of immigrants who came to the United States during or after the Famine years, while the memories were still fresh. More puzzling still, it was buried not only in the United States among Irish Catholics intent upon creating a new life, but in Ireland as well, where the survivors still had before their eyes ruined Famine villages and the telltale mounds of unmarked graves. Dublin-born poet Eavan Boland has written a wonderful poem called "The Emigrant Irish," which hints at a reason for the silence and the reason to break it:

> Like oil lamps, we put them out back,
>
> of our houses, of our minds. We had lights
> better than, newer than and then
>
> a time came, this time and now
> we need them. Their dread, makeshift example.
>
> They would have thrived on our necessities.
> What they survived we could not even live.
> By their lights now it is time to
> imagine how they stood there, what they stood with,
> that their possessions may become our power.
>
> Cardboard. Iron. Their hardships parceled in them.
> Patience. Fortitude. Long-suffering
> in the bruise-colored dusk of the New World.
>
> And all the old songs. And nothing to lose.

Like Eavan Boland, many Irish and Irish American people now have the confidence and courage to look back and learn. 1997 marked the hundred and fiftieth anniversary of Black '47, in many ways the worst year of the Famine. The anniversary let loose a flood of books, stories, songs, and conferences. Murals in Dublin Airport instruct travelers, and the Famine Museum in Strokestown, County Roscomman, opened in 1994 and now welcomes thousands of visitors every year. An Irish rock group calls itself Black '47; and in "Famine," Sinead O'Connor, who considers herself a contemporary keener, raps about precious food shipped out of Ireland while starving people looked on. Websites invite browsers to study drawings, cartoons, and newspaper articles from the Famine years. Forensic anthropologists are even beginning to excavate famine sites, including graves.

But before this flood, there was only a small trickle of articles and books, of which only one, Cecil Woodham-Smith's *The Great Hunger*, was widely read and roundly criticized. Woodham-Smith published her book in 1962, more than a hundred years after the Famine. There were, of course, thousands of contemporary newspaper accounts as well as stories written by survivors or taken down by oral historians; but these accounts were buried in archives, waiting for scholars and family members to bring them into the light.

How and why does a whole group of people bury a disaster so appalling that even when measured by the standards of the twentieth century it's almost unbearable to read about? I've read psychological, political, and literary explanations for this long silence. First, famine and disease were so pervasive and the number of deaths so overwhelming that no one kept track of how many men, women, and children died. Some say 1 million, some 1.5 million or more out of Ireland's population of 8.5 million. Most of the dead lie not in blessed and tended cemeteries but in unmarked graves or in fields and bogs where mass graves received each day's dead. They are invisible, nameless, voiceless. Those who survived, whether they stayed in Ireland or immigrated to the United States, were silenced in another way. They chose to turn a blind eye to the Famine in order to go on living. Irish historian Christine Kinealy writes of eloquent gaps in oral accounts: "The worst aspects of famine (of any famine)—stealing from each other, hoarding, feuding, nakedness, cannibalism, and agonizingly slow and obscene deaths—rarely appear, due to residual feelings of pain and shame." Like many other immigrants to the United States, my Irish ancestors must have blocked out the pain, guilt, and shame rather than passing it on to their children and grandchildren, beating it back every day in order to do that day's work of making a living and a life. They had to close the inner eye, the eye of memory, to scenes and experiences that would have turned them to stone or pushed them to suicide if they had looked intently, undefended by alcohol.

When survivors told the stories now kept in the Irish Folklore Archive, they often said that the Famine happened somewhere else, to someone else; it didn't happen in their family, their townland, their county. But even if the people had been willing to recount their experiences to sympathetic listeners, they probably would not have been able to find the words or the story form. Irish poet Brendan Kennelly calls Ireland "the grave of song" where "the desolation of the famine silenced the popular imagination for decades." In addition, many immigrants, my great grandparents among them, spoke Irish as their mother tongue, learning English in school or after they came to the United States. I can imagine that when you lose your first language, you also lose your ability to recount certain experiences, especially those laden with emotion.

Having learned what a heavy burden they carried, it's no wonder to me now that my great-grandparents put their hands over their mouths and carried their memories, unspoken, perhaps unspeakable, to the grave. In one way, it would be an act of mercy on the part of descendants like me to respect their chosen silence and stop turning up old graves. But the trouble with buried memories is that the next generations are heirs to a bitter residue without the corrective of history or the comfort of songs and stories.

Peter Quinn, another descendant of silent Irish parents, describes the pull of memories that I've felt for a long time but had no words for until now. He writes:

> Even amnesia, the absence of memory, cannot erase the imprint of the past. Recalled or unrecalled, memory is embedded in the way we love, hope, believe. Tamed, sublimated, suppressed, it will not disappear. It pulls on us like the moon's elemental urgings on the sea.

The title of Thomas Gallagher's 1982 history of the Famine is instructive. He calls his book *Paddy's Lament: Ireland 1846–1847— Prelude to Hatred.* Without the story of the Famine, terrible as it is, what I have from my Irish past is an incoherent tangle of nostalgia and pride and unexamined hatred; the shadows of alcoholism, mental illness, and anger; twisted attitudes towards law, authority, and government. I have the words and melodies to a hundred songs. But without the story of the Famine, my father and countless men like him seem inexplicable, maybe even pathological.

But learning and telling the story of the Famine isn't easy. As with any historical event, people have told many different versions during the years since 1845, when a strange fungus first reduced the Irish potato crop to a stinking mass not even the pigs would eat. To understand the Famine, in order to learn its lessons, it's important to sort out a complex mix of causes and responses, the fruit of deeply rooted prejudices. In fact, the Famine Museum in Strokestown hopes to instruct its visitors about present and future famines as much as or more than about Ireland's Great Hunger.

Mary Robinson, who was Ireland's president when the museum opened, has written that the Famine is "a human drama upon which we, as Irish people, place an enormous value, and by which we have been radically instructed."

But what are the lessons? While there is rough agreement about the facts, disagreement arises in the interpretation. Were the Irish peasants largely responsible for the disaster because of their folly in depending upon potatoes, dividing land into smaller and smaller parcels, and having very large families? Were they lazy, drunken, too dumb to fish or diversify their crops or their economy? Were the English benevolent colonial overlords, shouldering the burden of Ireland, were they bent upon exterminating the Irish Catholics, or were they something in between? Cormac Ó Gráda, a careful historical economist, describes Famine stories with tenacious roots in "folk memory" or "collective memory." These stories are, he says, a tangle of truth and half-truth: mass graves and brutal evictions alongside tales of vast amounts of Irish grain being shipped to England and Queen Victoria generously donating all of five pounds to famine relief. "For Ireland today," Ó Gráda says, "These stories are the Famine's most enduring legacy." Ó Gráda and other present-day historians are trying to correct the half-truths in order to find the truth. By analyzing potato production before the Famine, for instance, and comparing it to exports of grain, meat, and dairy products from Ireland to England during the five years of the Famine, Ó Gráda clearly shows that grain exports fell dramatically during those years. He also argues that even if all the food Ireland produced had stayed in the country, it couldn't have fed the 3.3 million Irish peasants who depended almost solely on potatoes for sustenance; another million or so whose diets included oatmeal, fish, and a bit of meat, in addition to six pounds of potatoes per day per person; and the pigs who also ate potatoes and whose fat sides paid the rent every year. This meticulous weighing of food produced and consumed softens to some degree accusations against the English government, which even during the height of the Famine refused to close Irish ports to English ships carrying food away.

Historians such as Christine Kinealy show that far from ignoring the Famine, the English were at first obsessed by it. It dominated parliamentary debate and British newspapers; for the first year or so, the government, the press, and the English people were honestly sympathetic and determined to help, to the tune of 10 million pounds from the government in grants and loans and another million in private donations. Historians have also examined the records of conscientious Irish landlords who came close to bankrupting their estates trying to feed their starving tenants. For example, the Marquis of Sligo of Westport put guns in his tenants' hands and sent them out to hunt in his private game park. Whatever they shot went into the big soup cauldron to be shared by all. Again, stories like this one diminish somewhat the charge levied both by the English and by Irish tenants: spendthrift, absentee landlords, all Protestant, most of them "planted" in Ireland in the seventeenth century by the English in an effort to claim Ireland for civilized Anglos, were responsible for the suffering of their tenants and damn well better deal with it. Most wastrel landlords, of course, didn't keep careful records for future historians to peruse. But beginning in the fall of 1847, when England dumped the full care of the starving Irish on the Irish landlords, almost all of them "dealt" with the problem by evicting hundreds of thousands of tenants, destroying their homes, and abandoning them to roads and ditches, disease-ridden workhouses, or coffin ships bound for Canada or the United States.

Historians have also studied the main political players in England and Ireland, such as the much-maligned and much-defended Charles

Trevelyan, undersecretary for the treasury, who played a leading role in shaping England's policy toward the Famine. Trevelyan was no Hitler bent on genocide; he was an earnest man who trusted in both divine providence and an unfettered market to correct all social ills, in this case, what he saw as Ireland's backward and self-devouring economy created by the moral failings of Catholics. His ideology freed his conscience to lay a million famine deaths at God's feet, a necessary sacrifice to bring about a greater good. In his words, the Famine was "a direct stroke of an all-wise and all-merciful Providence" to reveal "the deep and inveterate root of social evil." His one regret was that "the poor people . . . should be deprived of knowing that they are suffering from an affliction of God's providence." Some economic historians studying the aftermath of the Famine argue that it benefited Ireland, eventually cutting the population almost in half, eliminating the practice of subdividing landholdings, and ending the dependence on potatoes. One look at Ireland's burgeoning economy today can make Trevelyan's words in praise of Divine Wisdom seem prophetic. But rather than declaring him a prophet and the Famine a providential misfortune, I'd like to shine the light of history on well-off English and Irish people who were complicit in the sufferings of the Irish poor.

In common usage, the phrase *turn a blind eye* means that a person, group, or nation sees injustice or human suffering but chooses to shut their eyes to it. It's a willed blindness. Except for the most callous or corrupt, turning a blind eye requires a great effort to compromise one's sense of justice, decency, and compassion. This phrase accurately describes the stance of most members of the English government, most of the English people and the Irish gentry, and a large part of the English press during the worst years of the Famine. This particular *blind eye* took several forms. Some people looked intently, helped for a while, and then turned away, worn out by an excess of compassion. Others, though they knew what was happening, chose not to look; they stayed in England or in their Irish castles or opera boxes in London or Paris—anything to avoid peering into Irish hovels or being engulfed by the ocean of homeless paupers wandering the roads. Others were blinded by an entrenched hatred of Irish Catholics and still others by a treacherous combination of ideologies—religious, economic, social, political—cheering each other on like good old boys.

One thing is certain: even with one eye shut, no one in Ireland or England could truthfully say, "I didn't know what was happening." In fact, the international news media covered the Famine, as did every big newspaper in England and Ireland. Photography had been invented, and many photographs survive of the Irish "big houses" (many of which grew even bigger and more luxurious during the Famine) and of their genteel inhabitants, conspicuously at leisure. No one took photographs of the hungry Irish people. The *Illustrated London News*, which was sporadically sympathetic to the Irish poor, sent an artist named James Mahony to the west of Ireland and published his reports and his pencil sketches. In his drawings of soup lines, evictions, burials, beggars, and emigrations, only one person has a name: Bridget O'Donnell, a gaunt young woman who looks straight ahead, her arms around her children. Most paintings, drawings, news stories, and accounts by travelers to Ireland depict the mass of "mere breathing skeletons" but efface this man, this woman, this child, leaving them isolated in the loneliness of hunger.

Belated words can't ease that loneliness. But to know the Great Hunger, we have to imagine our way past the famine faces the twentieth century has made too familiar. We have to get past our own feelings of compassion fatigue. It might help to close our eyes and let our other senses shepherd the imagination.

Think of one woman; call her Bridget O'Donnell, from Kilrush in County Clare. Bridget's hands that know so much read the Braille of hunger on the dwindling bodies of her two surviving children. She checks anxiously for the fever burning in them. All around her are roofless and tumbled cottages, her own among them, where the fires have gone out, some of them after burning day and night for a hundred years. The neighbors are dead or turned out of their homes. Instead of the warm, bitter smell of turf fires, the smell of death is in the air—the rotten potatoes, the sick, the dying, the dead nobody has the strength to bury.

She hears silence. At first her neighbors sat on the fences and wailed for the stricken potato fields. One even made up a song, "A Thousand Farewells to the White Potato." They wailed for the dead and for family members leaving for the United States or England or Australia. Now no one sings, and most aren't even strong enough to beg or moan. Maybe the skylarks still sing at dawn as they rise on strong brown wings. Bridget doesn't listen for their song, or for the song of the little wrens, so much bigger than their bodies. Maybe the birds have died or left County Clare. She doesn't know.

Bridget's husband—let's call him Paddy—died before their last baby was stillborn. The cause hardly matters, there are so many possibilities: hunger, black fever, cholera, cold, despair. He'd farmed a couple of acres and fished the dangerous Atlantic. But Paddy pawned his nets and tackle to buy food in the early years of the Famine.

Bridget O'Donnell and her children have no home. She heard the shouts and the grating of crowbars on stone the night the bailiff pulled it down around them. Now they crouch at night in a ditch with a few pieces of turf leaning precariously overhead. Though the roads teem with people, her village is deserted. She has no family, friends, or neighbors to turn to. She feels the cold, the lash of rain and wind off the wild Atlantic. She feels hunger and terror for herself and her children. She feels the stones under her bare feet as she leads them to the Kilrush workhouse—her last hope—and to almost certain death.

But nobody wrote about Bridget in 1846 when her story might have made a difference. The influential *London Times* quickly got tired of telling the "tedious and wearisome . . . ten times told tale" of the Famine. On 11 November 1846, when the potato crop failed for the second disastrous year, the *Times* apologized to its middle-class English readers: "We can easily imagine that our readers are beginning to be a little tired of Ireland. If it is any consolation to them, or any apology for ourselves, we beg to assure them of a most entire sympathy with their fatigue."

In contrast, one of the people who looked compassionately at the suffering Irish was Frederick Douglass, an escaped U.S. slave who went on a speaking tour in Ireland in 1845 and 1846 to win moral and financial support for the abolition cause. The Cork *Examiner* reports that alongside the "influential men of the city" were the "suffering poor" who "thronged" to hear Douglass. The "influential men" must have been jostled by the throngs of "suffering poor" as they entered the lecture hall to hear Douglass talk about the evils of slavery in the United States. While they seem to have been blind to this irony, Douglass was not. He wrote to William Lloyd Garrison that he had seen many Irish people living in conditions worse than those of the meanest slave in the United States.

I don't think it's possible to understand the deeply rooted anger and sense of degradation many Irish Catholics brought with them to this country without looking squarely at this willed blindness and its consequences. The Irish peasants who survived the Famine—those from Strokestown or Sligo, Skibbereen or Rahana, Tipperary or Clones—my ancestors among them, did not and could not know extenuating facts and events; still less could they see beyond each day's hunger to a prosperous future. About half were illiterate. They got the news from neighbors or from speakers at nighttime meetings. They knew their country's brutal history, the English version recorded in the textbooks some of them read in school, the Irish version passed on in songs and stories; most of all, they knew what they saw, felt, smelled, tasted, lived. That knowledge, that "folk history," must have been what they brought with them to the squalid tenements of New York, Boston, Philadelphia, and New Orleans and eventually to the green fields of Leaf Valley, Minnesota. Here is a small part of that lived history, gleaned from reports by journalists, travelers, politicians, and the survivors themselves. It's not the whole story, but its rough outline forms a composite memory for the Irish Catholics who came to the United States after the Famine. It's a history my dad and most Irish Americans of his generation never heard, even though its thready blight reached into their lives.

Even before 1845, most Irish peasants knew yearly hunger and were always just scraping by. For instance, in County Donegal in 1837 there was one chair for every ninety people and one bed for every nine hundred. Two-fifths of Irish families, most of them very large, lived in one-room cabins about twelve by eighteen feet, made of turf or unmortared stones. But this famine was different from the forty preceding ones. It was Án Gorta Mór, the Great Hunger. The suddenness and virulence of the potato blight made it seem like a biblical plague, sent as punishment for grave sin. One day, the potato fields were green and flowering; they looked beautiful and promised a good crop. The next day, black spots appeared on the leaves. The plants withered, and the potatoes turned into a stinking, inedible mass. No one knew what caused the blight or where it came from, so there was no effective way to prevent its recurrence. In 1845 it destroyed a third of the crop; in 1846 the destruction was total. The potatoes were healthy in 1847, but hungry families had eaten the seed potatoes, and the crop was sparse—only one-sixth of what was needed. In 1848 the potato crop failed again, with partial failures in 1849, 1850, and 1851.

Peasants who had livestock ate their pigs, chickens, sheep, and horses. Those who didn't poached livestock and game. They ate dogs, cats, and rats, seaweed, nettles, and grass. They ate handouts of Indian corn imported from the United States and thin gruel served up at soup kitchens. Some say they ate the dead. When the food was gone, they starved to death or died of exposure in 1846 and 1847, the worst winter the west of Ireland had ever known. One description of starving children stands for the million: "Most pitiable was the appearance of the heads of these children, for as the hair thinned and then gradually left the scalp in patches, the almost translucent pallor of the skin exposed the cranium so that it appeared too insubstantial to prevent a poking finger from entering the brain. At the same time, as if some cosmic joke were being played on them, hair grew from their chin and cheeks, a thick sort of down from their forehead and temple." Predictably, travelers compared the children to chimpanzees. Charles Kingsley, an English clergyman and professor of modern history at Cambridge, was especially horrified that those chimpanzees were white.

Terrible diseases accompanied the Famine, all of them fiercely contagious and almost always fatal after days or weeks of anguish that family members could only watch, often from a distance. Starvation brought on scurvy and dropsy. The people abandoned wakes and funerals, those ancient rituals that link the living and the dead, and resorted to reusable coffins with hinged bottoms and mass graves for the dead and the all but dead. Some people died in ditches and fields and were eaten by starving dogs, pigs, and rats. One observer reports wresting a child's severed head from a dog.

Sometimes a whole family huddled in the back corner of their hut, closed the door, and died with some small scrap of dignity. One eye witness reports that "such family scenes were quite common, and the cabin was generally pulled down upon them for a grave." As one survivor said, "The Famine killed everything." Included in that *everything* are family members, certainly, but also music, ritual, celebrations, family loyalty, and communal solidarity. Sometimes fear and hunger killed even the love between parents and children as they fought each other to survive.

While Irish cottiers couldn't know how many tons of food were leaving their shores in English ships, they must have been enraged and finally driven to despair to see wheat, barley, oats, butter, eggs, bacon, fish, and millions of head of cattle bound for England or her colonies, sometimes in the same cattle boats that carried emigrants to Liverpool to begin their hazardous trip across the Atlantic. When they tried to stop the ships from leaving port, Trevelyan sent in two hundred additional troops to bolster the Royal Irish Constabulary and the fifteen thousand regular British troops already stationed in Ireland.

The Irish peasants must also have been aware of how inadequate and finally cynical and cruel—in practice if not in intent—the relief efforts of the English government were. The corn imported from the United States and elsewhere in 1846 and 1847 was not nearly enough to feed 4 million hungry people, many of whom could not afford to buy it at any price and especially not at prices controlled by landlords and the market. In 1846 the Earl of Dunraven in Limerick bought half a ton of corn and offered it to his starving tenants for two pence a pound, more than twice what a man could make in a day on a government work project, if he was lucky enough to have a job. Convinced that the Irish needed moral uplift more than they needed food, the English government organized public works, making the work so hard and the pay so low that only the truly desperate would apply. Still, in 1847, before England abandoned the works program, over seven hundred thousand men competed daily for eight to ten hours of back-breaking work for less than a penny. The projects were worthless by design, not the building of railroads or even the improvement of cropland, but rather breaking rocks to build what Eavan Boland calls "Famine Roads," "small, bitter trails in the woods, giving out into a nothingness."

In Black '47 as many as a million people lived in work houses, often called "slaughter asylums," where the well, the sick, and sometimes the dead were packed in together. Families were separated, and many of the workhouse inmates were orphans or children whose parents had been evicted or who had given up their land and their home, a requirement for admission. Late in 1847 when England turned over "the Irish problem" to the Irish landlords, the misery and evictions increased. Brendan Ó Cathaoir presents the bleak numbers: "Evictions peaked at 20,000 families—over 100,000 children, women, and men, in 1850. In 1847 there were almost 730,000 farms in Ireland; by 1851 the number had fallen to 570,000." In July 1847, 3 million people queued up daily for watery soup. Tens of thousands of tenants wandered the roads and stormed the gates of cities, which were closed against them. Whole villages and towns were deserted. County Monaghan, for example, lost 40 percent of its population. County Mayo lost one out of three to death or emigration.

People grieved as they watched their neighbors and then their children leave Ireland. Historians disagree about the willingness of the Irish peasants to leave their homeland, and the Irish still sing boisterous pub songs about going to California, where "instead of diggin' praties" they'll "be diggin' lumps of gold." Still, until the twentieth century there was no word in Irish for voluntary emigration. Irish speakers had only the word *deorai*—"exile." In December 1846, the Belfast *Vindicator* asked rhetorically, "What compulsion is stronger than that in which the alternative is starvation?" Whether by choice or compulsion, more than 2 million seized the escape route of emigration between 1845 and 1855. Most were desperately poor, and many were sick. Tens of thousands died in the slums of Liverpool before the ships ever sailed; many more died on the way or soon after they arrived in Quebec, New York, or Boston, where even before the Famine, more than half of the children died before reaching the age of five.

My great-grandparents were all children during the Great Hunger. Somehow, their parents kept them alive. I'll never know how they did it. Maybe they weren't among the desperately poor, owning enough land to raise cattle. Maybe their survival depended on someone else's death. But regardless of their situation, in that small, thickly populated country, there was no way to avoid knowing the suffering of their neighbors and the bald fact that not everyone in Ireland was hungry or even living frugally. Even the good Lord Sligo of Westport considered it a sacrifice to rent out his London opera box to help feed his tenants.

In April 1847, well-to-do women paid five shillings to watch paupers eat at the soup line of the French chef M. Soyer. The ladies even served them "with their own fair hands." The five shillings went to famine relief. The *Weekly Freeman's Journal* of Dublin commented bitterly: "Five shillings each to see paupers feed!—five shillings each to watch the burning blush of shame chasing pallidness from poverty's wan cheek!—five shillings each! When the animals at the Zoological Gardens may be inspected at feeding time for sixpence!"

The notorious Strokestown Castle, now the site of the Famine Museum, had underground tunnels through which the servants scuttled so that Lord Mahon and his guests never had to see them. But that doesn't mean that the servants were blind to the excesses of their lords.

The Famine was terrible, whether we look into the face of one woman or broaden our view to encompass a whole starving nation. But it was not an isolated tragic event. It was the culmination of eight hundred years of British colonial rule. Understanding the bitterness of Irish Catholic immigrants demands that we understand something of that history. While England was not responsible for the potato blight or for Ireland's dense population, she was responsible for economic, social, and political oppression that distorted the lives and spirits of the Irish Catholic peasants. The British found countless ways to convince them that they were stupid, lazy, barbaric, immoral, violent, and clearly unfit to rule themselves. The most sympathetic saw them as strong laborers able to endure hardship and hunger. Few Irish peasants ever saw themselves caricatured in the *London Times* or in *Punch* with brutal, apelike faces or looking more like their potatoes or their pigs than like their civilized English neighbors; still, the conditions of their lives taught them indelible lessons of English ethnic and religious bigotry and contempt for everything Irish, from the brogue, to "lazy" farming methods, to the uncorseted Irish women.

I said earlier that I went to Ireland half expecting to find that my grandfather James Faulkner was a Fenian. When I visited the place where Rahana, his townland, used to stand, I found the fading scars of imperialism criss-crossing the green land. Louth is one of the northernmost counties of the Republic of Ireland, bordering Armagh, a county in the present Northern Ireland. The names of villages and towns suggest that Irish Catholics and English or Scots Irish Protestants lived right next to each other. Rahana was next to Charlestown, Clonkeehan across the field from Gilbertstown,

Ballybaillie near Riverstown, and Kilcroney down the road from Tallanstown. Rahana was located in an area of great natural beauty, with rounded hills and wide green fields and flowers blooming in every season: primrose, pansies, holly, and azaleas giving way in spring to fuchsia, rhododendrons, and roses. A huge estate still stands there surrounded by high hedges and a beautifully symmetrical stone fence more than a hundred yards long. It's a private game preserve now, but when my grandfather was a boy, the land as far as the eye can see would have been the domain of an English or Anglo-Irish landlord, and my grandfather's Catholic parents would have been tenants or day laborers, with little hope of improving their lot.

In nearby Charlestown stands a stately church, deserted now, built by the Protestant Church of Ireland in the 1830s. When I first saw it, I assumed that prosperous and generous Protestants donated the money to build it. Later I discovered that from 1691 to 1870 all Catholics were obliged to pay tithes to support the established Church of Ireland. If they couldn't or wouldn't pay, the tithes were added to their rent, which the landlords collected. In 1833, for instance, tithes amounted to six hundred thousand pounds, $1.25 million dollars in today's currency. Catholic peasants like my ancestors built that church and many like it across Ireland and paid rent on the 5 million acres of farmland the Church of Ireland owned.

The church in Charlestown stands as a symbol not only of English religious bigotry but also of economic policies designed to impoverish the Irish and keep them poor. Its very existence depended upon laws the Irish had no hand in making but had to obey. It is understandable, then, that peasants who were turned out of their cottages by the "crowbar brigade" would vow to take their hatred of the English to the grave and beyond and to teach their children to do the same.

In 1801 the Act of Union made Ireland a part of Great Britain, but Ireland's few MPs and British sympathizers had very little political power. The vast majority of Irish peasants had no political voice at all. Because of literacy and property requirements, only a little over 1 percent of the Irish population could vote: 122,000 out of 8.5 million before the Famine, and only 45,000 in 1850. Of the millions of Irish Catholics who came to the United States between 1845 and 1885, few had ever cast a vote. While there were violent secret societies and many uprisings, the people had no legal way to bring about change. They also had no direct experience and no historical memory of a government having their best interests at heart. They had the opposite: a foreign government that for centuries aggressively exerted its will and in the Famine tragedy turned a blind eye to the suffering of millions. Irish Catholics didn't know what it was like to respect and obey laws they had helped make. In 1839, the French historian Gustave de Beaumont wrote about an Irish court he observed: "The judge and jury treat the accused as a kind of idolatrous savage, whose insolence must be subdued, as an enemy that must be destroyed, as a guilty man destined beforehand for punishment. . . . Who will be astonished that in Ireland this hatred of the law is universal?"

Sometimes sociologists point to the Irish as object lessons for the other large groups of immigrants to the United States, calling them the "ideal immigrants," the ones who, after a rocky start, melted smoothly into U.S. social, political, and economic life. But this success story ignores my father's parents and grandparents and the many like them who carried heavy baggage into the steerage of the ships that brought them here: hunger memories, for sure, but also the smoldering anger that comes from colonial rule and the leeching of self-esteem caused by what W. E. B. Du Bois calls "double consciousness." Du Bois was writing about African Americans, but his description of this chaotic inner state also fits Irish Catholic immigrants. Their conviction of their own worth and of the value of their religion, language, history, and culture was at war with the terrible suspicion that the colonizers might be right. Put into words, that internal quarrel might sound something like this: "The English call us bog-trotters, potato-eaters, lunatics, beggar-assassins who take English charity and spend it on guns. But we can sing and dance and tell stories. We work hard. We create. We have a long, varied, sometimes heroic, sometimes violent, always human history. Our children are beautiful and smart. Then why are we on the bottom and the English on the top?" How long can a people hold on to these opposite opinions of themselves, and what kind of fissures do they create in their minds and hearts?

Most of the Famine Irish who landed in the United States were sick, hungry, traumatized, and unskilled. In the shanty towns, slums, and "big houses" of New York, Boston, Philadelphia, and New Orleans, they encountered again many of the same prejudices they'd left behind. They also found the same poverty and diseases, as well as some new ones, such as yellow fever, to which they had no immunity. They were once again at the bottom of the social heap, fighting freed slaves for the dirtiest, hardest, most dangerous jobs at the lowest wages. Many men lived short lives, marked by disease, gang fights, alcoholism, family violence and desertion, and mental illness. In New Orleans in 1853 one Irishman out of every five died; during the Famine, the rate was only one in seven. In his article "Of Famine and Green Beer," John Leo writes: "Irish violence was often astounding. Bodies floated in New York City's East River almost every day. At one point, the city jail population was 90 percent Irish. Police vehicles that rounded them up were called 'paddy wagons,' the wagons that carried all the hopeless Paddys to their natural home. Cartoonists drew pictures of the Irish as crazed monkeys, and good citizens wondered about a permanently unfit underclass and the possibility of genetic inferiority." In the United States, too, the Irish met vicious anti-Catholicism embodied in the Know-Nothing Party and, because they were poor laborers—miners, textile workers, canal and railroad builders, drainers of swamps—they found exploitative employers and laws that failed to protect them. The difference was that in the United States, they were free to make a place for themselves in the political system.

Given their history, it doesn't surprise me that the Irish used legal means to improve working conditions for laborers and at the same time suspected the government and felt free to bend it to their purposes. Sometimes the same individual or organization worked both inside and outside the law. While the Irish certainly did not invent political corruption in the United States, they caught on fast. Almost all of the powerful Democratic political machines in big cities from New York to San Francisco were run by Irish bosses, of whom Chicago's Mayor Richard J. Daley was merely the most notorious. But they also became effective union organizers and crusaders for working people and farmers. Hundreds of thousands of Irish workers joined labor unions, which Irish immigrants or their children founded or led. Many were jailed for breaking laws they considered unjust and for demanding the right to speak, march, and unionize.

The obituary of my great-grandfather Dennis Maloney in the Alexandria, Minnesota, *Citizen* describes him as a lifelong Democrat, in Republican rural Minnesota, who rarely missed a county convention. The obituary also says that Dennis was "a true type of sturdy manhood—faithful, generous and noble in all his instincts, loving right, liberty and justice and hating cruelty, wrong and oppression in its every guise and form." These words might be a generous fiction created by the newspaper's obituary writer, but I choose to believe them; looking back, I see these qualities in my dad alongside his ready bending and breaking of laws.

Growing up in a family dominated by our dad's inconsistent values and actions, my sisters, brother, and I didn't know Irish history and had no way to learn it. North Dakota schools in the forties and fifties were as silent about the Famine as they were about the Japanese internment camp just down the road from Mandan and the injustices suffered by the Mandan, Hidatsa, and Arikara Indian tribes who lived near us. Lacking knowledge, we could only react to our dad's flouting of the law as children do, with love and fear, pride and shame, excuses and judgments, submission—often masking inner revolt—and outright rebellion against actions we knew were wrong. While I can't speak for my sisters and brother, for me, this research has been a chance to reflect on the hard lessons our dad's life has taught me and the equally hard lessons I've learned from the Great Hunger.

I learned to be outraged at injustice, especially that inflicted on "the little guys," and to feel responsible to challenge, change, and, if necessary, break unjust laws. The Famine Irish and their descendants stepped into a long, respected tradition in the United States of citizens whose consciences would not tolerate slavery, child labor, Jim Crow, segregated schools, taxes to support wars of aggression, torture and training for torture, and unfair immigration policies, to name just a few of the laws conscientious citizens, many Irish among them, have protested and sometimes changed. But I also learned that it's a short, slippery downward step from conscientious objection to unjust laws to the conclusion that the government itself is illegitimate and its laws not binding. As Tom Hayden says, many Irish Catholic immigrants decided that "if there was no hope for the redistribution of wealth . . . at least the Irish could redistribute the graft." There was a dark side to my dad's sometimes playful, sometimes serious breaking of the law, and even his fierce sense of justice. Though his generous heart always went out to children, he turned a blind eye on the damage his law breaking may have caused. Did the boy with the big firecrackers lose his eye? What happened when the Indian men—most of them alcoholics—came home to their wives and children drunk on hard cider? What did his law breaking do to us, his children, terrified, angry, protective, or split off from our own sense of justice and right?

Still, as I look back on my father's life, I find his unquestioning allegiance to Joseph McCarthy and the House Committee on Un-American Activities much more frightening than his breaking of laws. McCarthy's brand of Americanism certainly would have condemned my brother when he resisted the Vietnam draft and was ready to go to prison for his convictions—a decision my father didn't live to see. I've always wondered whether he would have been proud or desperately ashamed of his only son. For it is also a short and slippery step from a clear-eyed respect for elected government and its laws to an unquestioning adherence to them.

Blind devotion to law and the authority of government with its bolstering ideologies leads inevitably to injustice, as it did in England during the Famine. After making all possible allowances for individuals and groups in England and Ireland who worked heroically though futilely to fend off starvation, I dare not excuse the English and the Irish gentry for turning a blind eye to suffering. Many historians say that they were simply acting by their best lights and by the limited wisdom of the Victorian age. But at the very least they were guilty of what political philosopher Judith Shklar calls "passive injustice": "a form of injustice whose corrosive effects may be all the greater precisely because it passes for normality, for propriety on the parts of well-intentioned people (however mistaken or ill-advised.) Active injustice involves the breaking of rules but passive injustice may ensue from simply doing nothing, or from an over-zealous adherence to rules and accepted routines. In its most familiar forms, passive injustice is displayed by the apathy which enables citizens to turn a blind eye in the face of acute suffering and even matters of life and death."

It doesn't take much imagination for me to find myself in that description or in the averted faces of the people who saw the starving Irish and were more attentive to their own tender feelings than to the life and death struggle in front of them. It doesn't take any imagination at all to see men, women, and children dying of hunger and disease today. Their faces—twenty thousand of them a day—are right in front of me when I turn on the TV or open a newspaper. I dare not excuse the English and the Irish gentry, for if I excuse them, I will also excuse myself and my country for our own "passive injustice."

In *The Middle of Everywhere: The World's Refugees Come to Our Town*, psychologist and anthropologist Mary Pipher describes a silence like that of the Famine Irish in the immigrants from Somalia, Sudan, Iraq, Sierra Leone, Ethiopia, Bosnia, and several other countries who have come to Lincoln, Nebraska, since 1990, all refugees from famine and war. Pipher and other psychologists offered free therapy sessions to the newcomers, thinking that they would want to talk about their terrible experiences. Almost all of them refused the offer for a variety of personal and cultural reasons. But all needed emotional and spiritual healing; all needed to mourn their dead loved ones, many of whom lie in unmarked mass graves just like the Irish. Pipher and church leaders from Lincoln worked with representatives from each culture to create fitting memorial services. In contrast, there were no healing services for the mass of Irish refugees who struggled ashore in the nineteenth century and no way for them to lay their beloved dead to rest. It is too late to create a wake for the Famine dead. Important as remembering is, we risk being lulled into a new forgetfulness by memorials and belated apologies for wrongs done to and by our ancestors.

Among hundreds of beautiful, informative, or whimsical tourist stops in Ireland is one that doesn't make it into many guide books. It's a coffin ship sculpted by John Behan out of harshly twisted bronze, resting in dry dock at the edge of Clew Bay, near Westport, the good Lord Sligo's home. Skeleton bodies seem to be throwing themselves overboard. The three masts, without sails, reach toward heaven like three crosses or gallows, or maybe like the three-fingered hand of a prophet. The ship is a relic, never—please God!—to sail again from Ireland's shores. This Famine monument is shadowed by Croagh Patrick, Ireland's holy hill, which barefoot pilgrims climb every year on the last Sunday in July as they have for hundreds of years. They come to remember, atone, and implore. On the summit is a rough cross, newly planted, with this inscription: "In memory of all who died in Ireland through violence." Whether intentionally or not, these two monuments placed so close together suggest to me the final lesson of the Great Hunger. They suggest the inevitable links between hunger and violence and a new fleet of coffin ships carrying the fleeing poor. They say to me that violence, whether lawless or lawful, whether perpetrated by gangs, guerillas, or governments, whether armed with weapons or entrenched ideologies, creates many kinds of hunger—for food, a home, respect, useful work, self-determination, creativity. Unappeased, these hungers create another round of violence. Until we find a way to break that cycle, the Famine dead of many nations won't rest in peace, and their descendants, like my Irish ancestors, will bring to the United States corrosive hatreds more blinding than my father's physical blindness.

FIVE

Blind Faith

Not based on reason or evidence; unquestioning:
put blind faith in their leaders

WHILE THERE ARE certainly blind people who are
atheists or agnostics or who find God, religion,
and faith irrelevant to their lives, that was not true
for my father nor for the many blind people who have written
movingly about their struggles to believe in a loving and merciful
God. But I would not accuse any of them of having blind faith,
at least not in the conventional definition of that phrase. Like
most phrases containing 'blind,' *blind faith* is not positive. It
suggests stupidity, apathy, passivity. It describes people who lack
perception, wisdom, a healthy skepticism, and the backbone to
form their own convictions and obey their own consciences.

But for my father, as for many people both blind and sighted,
faith and the most radical questions seem to have coexisted. As
a boy and a young man, he attended Sunday Mass with his

family, mastered the Latin responses so he could be an altar boy, and later sang in the church choir, raising his true, resonant bass-baritone voice alongside the Germans and Poles in the Millerville, Minnesota, church. In the letters he wrote to my mother in 1936 and 1937, he often mentioned going to Mass and sometimes hearing "swell" sermons. When work kept him from church, he prayed the rosary. He assured Hattie that he was praying for her and for Sister Carlotta, her beloved oldest sister, who was a member of the Benedictine order in St. Joseph, Minnesota, and who was sick with tuberculosis. In the early days of their marriage, before they could afford a car, he and my mother walked more than five miles to Sunday Mass at St. Mary's Cathedral in Bismarck, from their house in the woods near the Heart River. They crossed a long car bridge over the Missouri River, the water brown and sluggish or ice covered far below them.

But that's not the man I remember, the man I prayed for every night of my childhood. Being Catholic was an essential part of my dad's Irish identity, a part he would never have renounced. But it now seems inevitable to me that his questions and resistance to authority should have extended to the authority of the Catholic Church, especially that exerted by the all-too-human priests and monsignors. In fact, I suspect that he inherited from his Irish parents and grandparents a fierce loyalty to Catholicism coupled with an equally fierce questioning of teachings or practices that seemed nonsensical or cruel to him.

This conflicted relationship to the Church is certainly rooted in Ireland's history as a colony of England, in England's efforts to wipe out "Papism," and in its refusal to die. The Catholic Church in every village, with its numerous feast days and rituals to celebrate life's passages, was the center of Irish social life. Many people, especially the men, followed Church regulations loosely. But after all those centuries of struggle, it would have been unthinkable for the vast majority to renounce the Church or fail to have birth, marriage, sickness, and death blessed by the Church's sacraments. In fact, being Catholic was one way for Irish peasants to resist British domination. It wasn't an easy way because of centuries of outright persecution followed by economic pressures. Until the twentieth century, almost the only way to prosper in Ireland was to join the Established Protestant Church. During the Great Hunger and even before, starving peasants could stay alive by taking handouts of soup from Protestant missionaries, sometimes given freely out of compassion, at other times only in exchange for conversion. *Souperism* was the popular word for this bartering of soup for souls, and *soupers* were the hungry Irish who traded their Catholic faith and, the Church would have said, their immortal souls to feed their families.

It wasn't only the English who believed that the Famine was God's way of punishing an immoral and improvident people. From the depths of their suffering, the Irish Catholics, too, began to fear that God was punishing them for some terrible sin: drinking, clinging to so-called "pagan" customs, and even wasting the plentiful potatoes in the years before the blight. After the Famine, some priests began to preach a harsh, sin-centered version of Catholicism to the demoralized survivors who stayed in Ireland.

But long before the Famine, I think that there must have been a buried anger fed by some of the logical but heartless teachings and practices of Catholicism. One teaching that the second Vatican Council quietly buried in the 1960s was the belief that infants who were stillborn or who died before they were baptized couldn't go to heaven. In traditional Catholic teaching, unbaptized infants were consigned to limbo. Limbo was a pleasant enough place but one where the unfortunate child would never see the face of God.

Like heaven and hell, limbo lasted forever. As the name implies, it was a cross between the two, a place of lukewarm happiness, where unbaptized babies languished just on the threshold of heaven. Unlike purgatory, a place of hopeful, cleansing suffering, there was no way out for the poor souls in limbo. I came upon two cemeteries for unbaptized children on a tourist map of tiny Achill Island off the west coast of Ireland. There may be similar cemeteries near every Irish town, and, since the teaching about limbo was universal, near Catholic cemeteries around the world. The children's cemeteries on Achill Island are almost inaccessible, poised near the cliff's edge high above the wild Atlantic. How many Irish babies slipped away before the priest arrived or before the parents could take them to church to be baptized? I wonder what that double tragedy would do to parents and what kind of fear and hatred of the Church this teaching could create in the hearts of mothers and fathers who looked into the pure eyes of their babies and then were forced to lay them to rest in unblessed ground, far from the village and the hominess of the family plot. Much worse than burial in an unconsecrated cemetery was the eternal fate of these babies. Instead of heaven, a place where all tears would be wiped away and all the lost and scattered reunited, babies who died "in the state of original sin" would spend their eternity in that bland and lonely place where they would never see God or their families. Who knows with what compassion or regret the priests delivered this bad news? It doesn't really matter, though, because there's no way to soften it for parents already grieving the loss of their child.

What do you do if leaving the Church is unthinkable, for in Ireland where else was there to go? How do you remain in an institution that claims to mediate the word and will of God, claims to be the guardian and interpreter of the Good News, claims to turn "darkness into light" in the brilliantly illuminated Book of Kells—claims all that goodness and wisdom—and then banishes your precious cold bundle to the company of the unredeemed?

Both in Ireland and in the United States, many children died at birth or soon after, especially during the Famine and in the following decades. It is likely that most families suffered this double loss or knew someone who had. My dad's grandparents, Dennis and Elizabeth Maloney, had eight children. Six of them grew to adulthood. One, Martin, died when he was a little over a year old and is buried in Seven Dolors Cemetery in Millerville. The eighth baby is a mystery. He was born like the rest in Leaf Valley and has a birthdate on a census form, but no name and no marker in the family plot. He is a baby consigned to limbo. Did the Maloney family keep the baby alive in stories? Did resistance begin to take root in my dad as he listened? I don't know. Whatever the cause of his questions about the Catholic religion, they became more and more numerous and, for me, more and more frightening.

By the time I was in grade school, and the implacable lessons of Catholicism had begun to take hold in me, Dad was attending Sunday Mass less and less often and then only when my mom or a kid begged him to go—at Easter, or for a first communion, confirmation, or graduation. He did that unforgivable thing: he openly questioned the authority of the Catholic Church, asking why he should go to confession to a priest whose sins all of Mandan was talking about or why we should eat fish on Friday when it was four times as expensive as the cheap hamburger that was the staple of our diet. I suspect that he questioned other Church teachings, ones he couldn't talk to his children about, like the ban on artificial contraception promulgated by a celibate clergy. Any kind of birth control, other than abstinence or the notoriously unreliable "rhythm method," was deemed mortally sinful because it violated the natural end of marriage and sex—the conception and bearing of children. Besides, said the Church's faith, any children God sends, God will take care of. But my dad saw his wife, exhausted and sick as she brought home her sixth child in seven and a half years; he saw himself, an aging father, doggedly trying to meet the needs of all those children. He probably knew that some of them were getting lost in the shuffle and didn't know what to do about it. When that sixth baby came home, Jeanne, who was four years old, hid behind the stove, expecting her mother to come and find her. For surely Mama had missed her as much as she had missed Mama. But my mother didn't find her; she may not even have missed her in the crowd. She sat wearily in the old rocking chair and nursed the new baby, while Jeanne crouched in her hiding place.

With the changes of Vatican II, the Church came around to my dad's way of thinking on some of these issues. But in the forties and fifties, I couldn't know that change would happen. As my father's faith in the Catholic Church seemed to fade, mine grew, but mine truly was the blind faith of someone afraid to question but quick to ferret out sin. Every night we knelt down beside the bed, eyes tight shut, hands folded, little girls in crisply ironed pajamas, even those made beautiful by my mother's touch. We repeated the words after her: "Angel of God, my guardian dear, to whom God's love commits me here." "God bless Grandma, Sister Carlotta, and all the poor people." "Make Daddy's eyes better." Later, I added my own plea to my mother's gentle prayers: "Bring Daddy back to the Church." By that I meant that I wanted him to follow all the rules so that he wouldn't die and go to hell for all eternity. Limbo wasn't a possibility for him.

I had been taught the commandments by the well-meaning Benedictine sisters in St. Joseph's grade school, but the lessons that really stuck came in sixth grade when a new priest I'll call

BLIND FAITH

Father Peter Olson came to town. He had been a Lutheran before he converted to Catholicism, a religion that apparently satisfied his desire for certainty. The priesthood was for him the essence of spiritual perfection and power. A cross between Mephistopheles and Bishop Fulton J. Sheen, he was a good-looking man with burning eyes and a flamboyant preaching style that brought to story-starved Catholics all the drama, gore, and vengeance to be found in the Bible, but none of the tender love. (Being Catholic, most of us had never read the Bible on our own. Protestants did that. We Catholics went to endless Requiem Masses, living rosaries, and Stations of the Cross, learned from the Benedictines to sing Gregorian chant, and memorized permutations of sins from our examination of conscience booklets.) Father Olson wore a long black cape and paced in front of the church, telling his rapt congregation stories of Jonah and his whale, Samson and Delilah, David and Bathsheba, Sodom and Gomorrah.

Ignoring the stories of mercy and forgiveness, Father Olson brought us face to face with a God of wrath, far above us yet watching our every move for the smallest punishable offense. Besides delivering long Sunday sermons, he came regularly to the grade school classrooms. He had us memorize the books of the Old Testament for prizes of glow-in-the-dark crucifixes and Virgin Mary statues. He also had each of us bring a small assignment notebook. Then he dictated words for us to copy down and live by: "One mortal sin is enough to send my soul to hell. Only I can choose to commit a mortal sin. God does not send my soul to hell, I send my soul to hell." He taught us hundreds of ways to commit mortal sins, some of them the very things my dad was doing or not doing.

The kids with common sense or a healthy dose of skepticism, who ignored most of what grown-ups told them, shrugged off Father

Olson's fire and brimstone view of God and religion. My brother and several of my sisters were among them. I wasn't so lucky or so brave. By the end of sixth grade, I had won the lurid phosphorescent crucifix, but the beautiful world had become a place of doom. There was no safety anywhere—not in books or conversation or the privacy of my own mind and feelings. In church, the grain in the polished wood of the pews in front of me turned itself into a long-faced version of Father Olson, watching, watching, God's wrath come down to earth.

I shouldn't have believed anything Father Olson said, but I did, believed it about myself and, much worse, believed it about my father. Only my dad's death almost fifteen years later freed me in a flash from blind faith in these lessons of sin, guilt, and damnation. My novice director at St. Benedict's Monastery, her face anguished, brought me the shocking news that my dad, whom I hadn't seen in almost a year, had died suddenly of insulin shock. My first reaction was grief, then a flood of gratitude: oh, now he isn't blind anymore. My second reaction was the clenching fear that he was in hell, sent there for all the so-called sins he had committed. My third reaction was a conviction that hasn't wavered. In that moment, I threw overboard pretty much everything Father Olson had drummed into my head about sin and guilt. I knew and loved my father, this good man. If he wasn't in heaven, I would have nothing to do with that place or its black-caped guardians.

In the past few years I've read numerous memoirs written by people who, like my dad, went blind at some point after they had experienced the great joys of sight. What amazes me most about those memoirs is each person's eventual acceptance of blindness. For many people, it is faith in a loving and always present God that makes such stunning acceptance possible. In *The Planet of the Blind,* Stephen Kuusisto describes an affirmation of faith among his blind friends: "Recently I was up late with a group of seven blind men and women. Our tears flowed together like the pitch that binds the boards in a wooden boat. Each of them had lost their loyal and life-affirming guide dog to cancer or old age. So what is faith? One stricken woman who was sitting alone in a corner of the room suddenly said that God only gives you the burdens you can carry. There was a murmur of assent from the others."

These people were helped through blindness and the desolation of death by a God as loyal as a seeing-eye dog, who doesn't—or can't—remove the burden of blindness but who is reliably there to help them carry it and to lead them around the obstacles of despair. The psalmist sings, "Though I walk through the valley of the shadow of death, I fear no evil, for your rod and your staff are with me," naming layer after layer of darkness, through which the good shepherd—or maybe the good sheepdog—leads each person.

My dad never came close to accepting his blindness as part of God's loving plan, but I would not call him a faithless person. His early letters to my mom are filled with a quiet, taken-for-granted faith in God and prayer. In one letter he wrote, "Honey light a candle every Sunday and I will do the same and I think every thing will be alright with [the] help of God." In those days, he didn't flaunt his faith or rationalize it, though even then, doubts and questions crept in. After a three-week hospitalization for flu, he wrote a despairing letter about his fear that Hattie would give up on him and find someone who was more of a man: "I am afraid you will get discouraged and not care what happens but I am praying for you all the time. But some time prayers don't help and especially mine." Then marriage blessed him with everything he had been praying for: a wife he loved and who loved him, a succession of little girls and then a son, a life that was hard and good and always hopeful, and finally an end to the loneliness of his transient life. Every night of his life, no matter how long and hard the day had been, he knelt down by the bed and prayed silently to a God he must have hoped was still awake and listening. I don't know what words he said, and I can only guess at what he prayed for. But as the years went by and his eyesight diminished, perhaps the scales fell from his eyes, and he saw clearly that his prayer had not and would not bring him the simple favor he asked for: "Lord, I want to see." In the Gospels, Jesus was always moved by compassion and hurried to touch and open blind eyes. My dad may have wondered what he had done or not done that God didn't answer his prayer. Maybe it was his own fault because his faith was shaky and riddled with doubts. Jesus often asks his blind petitioners, "Are you confident I can do this?" When they answer, "Yes, Lord," Jesus says, "Because of your faith it shall be done to you." But if Dad's faith was shaky, my mother's was steady and sure. On the bulletin board in her kitchen, where she could pray them every day, she had these words:

> I believe in the sun
> even when it is not shining.
> I believe in love
> when I feel it not.
> I believe in God
> even when God is silent.

Maybe God wouldn't answer the prayers of a skeptic like him, but what about the prayers of his faith-filled wife and his children?

In his reflections on faith, Stephen Kuusisto writes: "I wish I could console people. I find myself thinking about Jesus. Why did he cure the blind in his lifetime, rewarding their faith before the unbelieving multitudes? Now he's silent on the matter. But I've found that I can't live without faith; still its inexplicable rules keep me awake, and I'm more than a little angry." I think that Dad, too, was more than a little angry at God and split between faith and doubt, afraid to believe and afraid not to believe. He would have understood a prayer called "Disability: A Lament," which asks why a good God would hold out the gifts of sight and then snatch them away:

Creating God:
You made the sky,
clouds of purest white,
with rays of fuchsia and orange and magenta at sunset,
and faces dear with the smiles of loved ones.
Today thousands were born without sight;
thousands more lost vision because of injury or disease.
And it was evening and morning of another day.
Did you call this Good?

But I don't think he ever stopped hoping and praying because he was praying not just for himself but for his beloved children. In fact, I now believe that faith was part of his resistance to blindness. My dad never heard of DNA or genes and didn't know the name or nature of his disease. He sometimes said he had "nerve blindness," without understanding what this broad diagnosis meant for him and his children. It wasn't until the 1970s, some years after my dad's death, that researchers at the University of Michigan mapped RP's inexorable path through several generations of our family. We learned that because of its particular familial pattern, my brother escaped; all six girls are carriers who can pass on the condition to their children and who might get more or less severe symptoms later in life. My dad didn't know that, but he knew that it was no coincidence that his grandmother, mother, brother, and several nephews were visually impaired or blind, and that three of my sisters had obviously inherited his extreme nearsightedness and wore heavy glasses from the time they were four. Coreen has told me that after her yearly eye exam, Dad always asked her if her eyes were better or worse and was sadder each year at the ominous news. If my father had accepted blindness as part of God's loving plan for him, he would have been accepting it for his daughters and their children. Against this fatalism, he set the resistance of his faith—in God, in medicine, in any straw he could grasp.

I don't know what my dad believed at the end of his life. When he was sixty-three, he almost died of complications of diabetes and a doctor's clumsiness. He was in the hospital for several months and came home tired and old. From then until he died seven years later, he went to church with my mom faithfully every Sunday. Maybe he was grateful for the miracle of life. Maybe he was afraid of death and judgment. Maybe he had simply given up on his questions. He once said that he had lived his hell on earth. He was surely talking about his blindness, but also about the growing sense of failure and suspicion that came with it for him.

Many kinds of faith are necessary for a full, rich, adventuresome life. Almost every sphere of human experience calls for a kind of faith analogous to religious faith, and many of them can accurately be called "blind faith," if we're willing to revise our understanding of that phrase. For faith is, by definition, a belief in what we can't see, often in the face of contrary evidence, whether that something or someone is God, democracy, human goodness and decency, science, or medicine. For the blind, the sighted, and everyone in between, all faith is blind faith.

It's true that blind people have to have faith in all sorts of things that sighted people don't have to believe because they can see, most basically, open space and solid ground. Blind people must depend on patterns, those built into the physical world by nature or tacit human agreement (stair steps, city blocks, curbs) or those they themselves create to make their corner of the world more predictable. John Howard Griffin, for example, learned to navigate his room by the sound of his radio, and Sally Wagner begged her overly helpful visitors not to put her kitchen utensils in places where she'd never find them again. My dad arranged his tools just so and depended on us to keep cupboard doors shut and the furniture in its familiar places. Predictability must be seductive for blind people, tempting them to stay on familiar ground rather than venturing into foreign terrain. Dad succumbed to that temptation as his vision waned, staying home where his feet could follow the rough concrete sidewalk from our house to our market and back, day after day. In contrast to the adventuresome life he had lived as a young man, Dad chose a world that was familiar, safe, small. His need to draw a protective circle around himself and his family grew stronger as he aged, until even his songs changed. Mona, his youngest daughter, never knew the man whose brash, defiant songs flung a challenge at the universe. He sang a different kind of song for her. A year before he died, the Australian pop-folk group the Seekers hit the top forty with "A World of Our Own." Dad listened to the radio for hours every day, memorizing songs whose words and melodies he liked. He loved this one. Walking from the market to the house, hand in hand with Mona, after a long day of dealing with "the public," as he called his customers, they sang together:

Close the door, light the light, we're staying home tonight
Far away from the bustle and the bright city lights.
Let them all fade away, just leave us alone,
And we'll live in a world of our own.

When they reached the haven of our house, where every inch and person was familiar, and no curious or critical eyes were watching him, he and Mona sang:

GOING BLIND

We'll build a world of our own that no one else can share.
All our sorrows we'll leave far behind us there,
And I know you will find there'll be peace of mind
When we live in a world of our own.

Oddly and sadly, that constricted world isn't a safe place; it's small and fragile in comparison to the threatening world outside. Eventually the threats, real and imagined, cross over and inhabit the mind of the blind person. To face down that fear, many blind and visually impaired people refuse to stay home. They place their faith in canes, dogs, and the good will of strangers. They head out into the noisy upheaval of Los Angeles, New York, or Paris. They even venture out in Lhasa, Tibet, whose streets are a treacherous jumble of cars, mopeds, unfenced construction sites, and potholes, some of them several yards deep and filled with water.

Or, if they're like Erik Weihenmayer, they climb mountains. In describing the sheer audacity of Weihenmayer's attempt to climb Mount Everest a *Time* magazine reporter wrote that the lack of pattern, rather than hypothermia, oxygen deprivation, and ice, was the greatest obstacle:

> But in the Khumbu icefall, the trail through the Himalayan glacier is patternless, a diabolically cruel obstacle course for a blind person. It changes every year as the river of ice shifts, but it's always made up of treacherously crumbly stretches of ice, ladders roped together over wide crevasses, slightly narrower crevasses that must be jumped, huge seracs, avalanches and—most frustrating for a blind person, who naturally seeks to identify patterns in his terrain—a totally random icescape.
>
> In the ice fall there is no system, no repetition, no rhyme or reason to the lay of the frozen land.

BLIND FAITH

What made Weihenmayer's feat possible? Certainly, it was his courage and his impressive mountaineering skills. But without his faith in his climbing partners and their answering faithfulness, he would have been doomed to spend his life on flatland. He dedicates *Touch the Top of the World*, his account of his mountaineering adventures, to all those people "who have never hesitated to connect their lives to mine." That rope of faith binds them together in mundane and spectacular ways. His partners had to be willing to "grump" Erik, that is, take him to the bathroom in howling blizzards high up on the mountain side; Erik had to be willing to be "grumped." When Erik and Chris Morris were climbing Mount Aconcagua, the highest peak in the Andes, a screaming gale drowned out the verbal directions that usually served as guides. For hours, Chris whistled into the gale to keep Erik climbing on the trail rather than heading toward and over a cliff. On another mountain, Chris guided Erik over a nine-foot crevasse by describing how to jump, how to land on the narrow ice ledge on the other side, and what the river, rocks, and glacier far below would do to him if he missed that ledge. Chris repeated cheerfully, "Make it a good one . . . because if you fall, you'll definitely die." Erik made the jump and later reflected: "There are moments in our lives when we can move forward in small increments, increasing the challenge bit by bit, but there are other times when security is merely an illusion, when we must summon our courage, gather up our past skill, and proceed by the power of sheer faith. To this day, I cannot explain how I triggered the circuits that enabled my legs to crouch, my body to lean forward over the abyss, and then my legs to spring, so that I launched across, through the roar of the river and the mist that rose up like cold frost." That was a spectacular leap of faith, but at every moment of every climb, Erik has to believe that his companions are people of good will who won't simply walk away.

GOING BLIND

After that leap and an arduous climb, Erik said jokingly to Chris, "Morris, you better not be getting any ideas to leave me here on this godforsaken mountain." To which Chris answered, "What could you do about it if I did?"

Faith is a gift forced upon blind people, who, by necessity, understand it in an immediate, almost physical way. But it is surely illusory to assume that only the blind must live by faith, if not in God then in science and medicine, human capacity and goodness, the endurance of the universe and its species. None of these is certain, and many are downright doubtful. All require a leap of faith with no guarantee that the ground on the other side of the abyss is solid enough to bear our weight. They demand that we rope ourselves to other fallible humans, all of us whistling into the wind.

"Seeing is believing," a denial of faith that echoes the Doubting Thomas of the Gospels, sounds confident and defiant, but it's not a trustworthy guide to life. Individuals, communities, and nations make daring leaps of faith all the time. Unless we agree to settle for radical mistrust and cynicism, we need to put our lives in human hands, believing they are trustworthy, that is, *faithful.* Barring round-the-clock surveillance by a very private eye, how does anyone know her or his spouse is faithful? Treaties between nations and the whole web of civic and financial interactions depend upon faith. The state of Minnesota gives me a license to drive, believing that I will obey traffic laws and won't drive drunk; and I have to believe the same about other drivers, as I pull into the blind spot of an eighteen-wheel semi, going seventy.

Placing ourselves in the hands of Western science, medicine, and technology, for all its hard proof and rigorous testing, requires countless acts of faith. Any example will do. Recently, I let a retinal specialist inject a drug into my right eye, hoping that it would slow down or cure the thickening on the macula. How many acts of faith did it take for me to open my eye and sit silent and still while the needle slid in? I can count them, starting with the doctor. I have to believe that he really has all the prestigious degrees named in the diplomas on his wall, that he's right about this treatment, that his hands are clean and an infection won't start in my eye and rage through my body. I have to believe that he's a man of integrity, sobriety, intelligence, compassion; that he's not hungover or preoccupied or deeply upset on the day he holds the needle and breaks the surface of my eye; that his hands are as steady as God's hands holding the precious world. I could go on. There are the scientists and drug companies that produced the drug and the medical equipment makers responsible for the needles and syringes. As we know, all of these people are sometimes guilty of accidental or deliberate malpractice and even fraud. Yet I signed the consent form, as millions of people do every day in our clinics and hospitals. If I had thought or questioned or researched my way through all those acts of faith, I'd never have gotten around to having the injection or any medical treatment. This certainly requires faith, if not blind, then visually impaired. My brother, Dennie, calls the American Medical Association and the Federal Drug Administration a "bunch of crooks." He trusts only a few of them. Yet, when his first grandchild was born with a hole in her heart and a defective pulmonary artery, her parents put Oceana Dawn—their sea of faith, their daybreak, their world—into the hands of surgeons. Faith like this is forced upon us over and over in our human lives, or maybe it's granted to us as a gift, as it is to blind people.

Some people would say that what I've described isn't really faith but rather a modified knowledge based on past experience. But both personal and communal history are jagged with the shards of broken faith. The world is full of people who willingly dupe the sighted and the blind and send them to their deaths. During World War II, for example, Jacques Lusseyran was a leader in the French Resistance. He was blinded by an accident when he was eight, yet the other members of his underground group trusted him, a sixteen-year-old, to screen all potential recruits. His intuition, his sense of treachery or truthfulness, was, as he says in his memoir, "infallible, or nearly." That *nearly* brought disaster. One of the recruits to Les Volontaires de la Liberté gave the names of everyone in the resistance group to the Gestapo. Almost all of them were captured, imprisoned, and tortured. Some, like Lusseyran, were sent to Buchenwald. Only a handful survived. One of them was Lusseyran, who wrote about this betrayal in *And There Was Light*. He experienced the worst that humans can do to each other, yet, astoundingly, his faith in God, his friends, himself, and life survived this human treachery. Moreover, his faith freed him to love and comfort the other prisoners. As he says, "I was carried by a hand. I was covered by a wing. . . . I could try to show other people how to go about holding on to life."

We've all suffered small and large betrayals, yet we continue to make treaties, pacts, covenants, vows, and promises that we intend to keep and expect others to keep. We continue to conceive and rear children, plant trees, teach—all ancient acts of faith. We know now, of course, how the sperm and egg come together to make a child, how a seed or seedling becomes an apple tree, and even a little about how people learn from each other. But the future of the human race, of plant species, and maybe of life on earth is as uncertain as heaven. Faith in the basic goodness of life and the friendliness of the universe seems to be essential for unconditional love. In times of high infant and child mortality, mothers quietly warn each other not to love their babies too much, lest their hearts be broken over and over by early deaths. In every age, we don't know whether there will be a future time in which the child we conceive will delight in apple blossoms, bite into an apple's crisp flesh, make pies and press cider, learning these skills like so much else from previous generations. Yet only the most despairing among us gives up entirely on the unseen and unseeable future. A young character in "I Stand Here Ironing," one of Tillie Olsen's great short stories, tells her mother she isn't going to study for the next day's tests because "in a couple of years when we'll all be atom-dead they won't matter a bit." She believes it, her mother thinks sadly, but most of us don't, as we put our faith in antiproliferation treaties, global accords to control pollution and the destruction of plant and animal species, and international pacts of many kinds.

I can't untangle the knot of suffering or death for myself or anyone else. I don't know anymore than my dad did why God seems to answer some prayers and ignore others. But I learned belatedly from him to be true to my questions, even though they destroy my serenity, and to resist answers that crumble under the pressure of daily life. Many of the memoirs of blindness I've read are stories of radical faith. Like my mother, the men and women who wrote them are not mouthing untested platitudes or using faith as a ready-made excuse for passivity or mute acceptance. Eric Weihenmayer, John Hull, John Howard Griffin, and Jacques Lusseyran all came through not only blindness but many other kinds of suffering: the death of parents, chronic pain, paralysis, betrayal, war. For them faith is a frayed rope that sometimes breaks on the jagged rocks, and sometimes holds.

SIX

Blind Prejudice

Performed or made without the benefit of background information that might prejudice the outcome or result: *blind taste tests used in marketing surveys.* To deprive of perception or insight: *prejudice that blinded them to the merits of the proposal.*

I N ANOTHER PUZZLING contradiction, the language tells us that blindness can metaphorically describe either the absence of prejudice or its glaring presence. Lady Justice is often pictured with a blindfold over her eyes, holding a balance in her outstretched hand. This image embodies the ideal of justice that can't be bought or sold. She can't see the people coming to her asking her to weigh conflicting claims and make a decision. She doesn't know if one is rich and influential and the other poor and helpless. She can't see a surreptitious bribe held out to her. She simply stands there, listening and waiting for the evidence on one side to shift the balance. Supposedly, a blind man or woman would make a good judge, perhaps the only unprejudiced judge. But the definitions of *blindness* and *prejudice* overlap at several points, and the inability to make clear, informed judgments is part of one definition of 'blindness.' 'Prejudice' is "irrational suspicion or hatred of a particular group, race, or religion"; a *blind opinion* is one that is "undiscriminating, for which no reason can be given; not based on fact, usually total and unquestioning." In fact, 'blind prejudice' is so common that a Google search revealed more than 5 million entries. But that common phrase doesn't tell us anything at all about blindness and not much about prejudice. Folded into 'blind prejudice' are a couple of questionable assumptions. The first is that there's a kind of prejudice that's not blind, a kind that is deaf or mute, let's say, or maybe even discriminating, reasonable, and based on fact, and, therefore, justifiable. Another assumption is that prejudice comes from not being able to see clearly or at all the group or individual standing in front of one. Of course, this phrase uses 'blind' figuratively to suggest that the prejudiced person's mind is darkened by ignorance or hatred.

In my father, I saw both the presence and the absence of prejudice. It has taken me most of a lifetime to understand his contradictory attitudes and actions and to acknowledge their stubborn residue in my life. That search convinced me that blind people are neither more nor less prejudiced than people who can see and that seeing, whether with physical or mental eyes, doesn't necessarily erase prejudice. On the contrary, sight often creates or reinforces prejudice.

Nowadays, it's fashionably liberal and, with gambling casinos on Indian reservations doing good business, even lucrative to claim kinship with some Indian tribe or other. In the North Dakota of the 1940s and 1950s, that certainly was not the case. Indians, or "those damn Indians," were in the same category as "niggers," "thieving gypsies," Jews, and "the dirty Japs" who were interned during World War II in Fort Lincoln, near Bismarck. All of those epithets were familiar parts of my family's vocabulary. I heard them from classmates and customers in our store. I heard them from my dad.

Yet when I remember my childhood, I remember a colorful array of people coming to our store and hanging around to talk with him. There were the Kellys and Murphys and Maloneys of his boyhood come to visit and the German-Russian and Bohemian Kautzmans, Schmidts, Kalvodas, and Brychtas, who made up most of the population of Mandan and surrounding towns. But there was also Abe Tolshinski, one of the very few Jewish people in our area, and a tall, husky black man with a big ring on his finger who joked with my dad and even with me on his many visits to buy watermelons. (Everyone bought watermelons from my dad; I learned much later that associating black people with watermelons is now an unrepeatable stereotype.) There was the caravan of gypsies who camped one summer on our land. I remember a sleek, dark-haired man who tap-danced on our front porch and a little girl with a piece of red velvet wrapped around her waist as a makeshift skirt. When she tried to dance like the sleek man, I was shocked to see that she wasn't wearing underpants but envious of her casual freedom. There was Mr. Echohawk, an Indian engineer who came to Mandan from Oklahoma to help build the oil refinery south of town. He needed credit to buy groceries until he got established in town and got it from my dad. Dad got word that the Mandan barber he'd been going to for years had refused to cut Mr. Echohawk's hair. Dad told us he'd never go to that barber again, and he never did.

My brother, Dennie, told me a story I'd never heard before. One day a black man walked down busy Highway 10 carrying a gas can. We had two red Texaco pumps in our yard, another of my dad's dogged efforts to find something to sell that would improve our finances. The man said he'd run out of gas five miles east, near the long bridge that spans the Missouri between Mandan and Bismarck. Dad filled the five-gallon can, and the man paid for the gas and was ready to walk back to his car carrying his heavy load. This was in the early fifties, when hitchhiking was not dangerous, and people readily stopped to pick up unfortunate strangers. But not a black stranger, not even a black neighbor.

As my brother tells the story, Dad asked the man how he got to the store and how he planned to get back. "I walked," he said. Did my dad know he was black? Probably, given his alert ears tuned to the rhythms of voices. Or maybe my mom whispered something to him.

"Ma, get the car," Dad said. And to the man, "We'll give you a lift." They went out together, leaving the store in the care of several wide-eyed children, something else that was safe in the fifties.

This story is full of mystery: What was that ride like, the blind man, his blond wife, and the black man together in the 1938 Plymouth coupe? Did they talk? Of course. My father talked to everyone. Why did my father perform this gracious, generous act? Did he understand swiftly that this man was an outsider in bigoted North Dakota as he felt himself to be? Was this an act of defiance? Did his strong Irish anarchic streak lead him to break not only laws but social mores as well? Did he want people to see this odd assemblage? Did he want his children to know that this was (as he would have said) the "white" thing to do?

In these and many other instances, did my father's blindness free him to know the person before he leapt to judgments based on color, ethnicity, religion, or physical attractiveness? Other blind people have told stories suggesting that they had this blessed freedom. John

BLIND PREJUDICE

Howard Griffin, the famous author of *Black Like Me,* was blind for about ten years as the result of a Japanese bombing raid during World War II. In *Scattered Shadows,* his journal of those years, he tells a moving story about a taxi driver named Wooly who often drove him from his farm in the Texas countryside to Fort Worth. On the first trip, Wooly seemed delighted to learn that John was completely blind. On a later trip he asked how John imagined the people he met and what mental picture he had formed of Wooly. John told him that he judged people by the way they acted and that he knew from Wooly's many blundering kindnesses to him that he had a good face. Again, Wooly was delighted. He said, "Boy, I don't know how you do it." Then Wooly disappeared. John learned from his supervisor that Wooly lived alone in a skid-row hotel with neither family nor friends and that he'd lost his job, as he always did, because of his nasty disposition. Finally, a fellow cabbie told John that Wooly was "uglier'n sin," with a terrible scar that twisted his face and made him repulsive to most people who met him. He answered the disgust he saw on the faces around him with anger, hatred, and complete loneliness. Griffin reflects: "This explained his jubilation that I could not see, that I could not see him as others had, but that I saw beyond his scar just as he had seen beyond my blindness. All those with whom I had spoken implied that I really did not know Wooly. But I was sure then that I was the only one who did. With me, he had been like any other man; with me, he knew that his face could not blind me to the quality of his heart." As Griffin's story suggests, blind people by necessity have to get to know people by a slower process than the speed of light waves bouncing off a face and hitting the retina. They have to depend on a voice, a conversation, and sometimes the report of a sighted person to know the supposedly crucial facts about the people they meet.

I'm sure, then, that blindness sometimes prevents swift leaps to judgment. But my father's contradictory words and actions convince me that prejudice is much more complicated and pervasive than it at first seemed to me and that blindness is no defense against it. It slides in through closed eyelids, bypasses ruined retinas, and imprints itself directly on the brain and then the heart. The United States is an intensely visual culture with a prejudice in favor of sight; this sometimes leads us to assume that vision is the most important or even the only way to learn. But teachers are becoming increasingly aware that we humans have many ways of knowing. All of us pull in accents, dialects, smells, tastes, the soft flesh or calluses on the hands we shake; and we judge, based on the thousand traces that history has left on every one of us.

Alongside my dad's generosity and apparent liking for an intriguing array of unacceptable people was the deep scorn he felt for whole groups of people—felt and tried to pass on to his resistant children. Those scorns and hatreds came from his Irish parents and grandparents, his place in the society of the thirties, forties, and fifties, and the political tensions and animosities in the United States, especially during World War II and the Cold War.

In addition to the English, the traditional enemies of the Irish, there were the Japanese and black people, whom he disliked and distrusted in general even though he befriended individuals from both groups. And then there were the German Russians or, as they call themselves now, the Germans from Russia. We learned from our dad little but disdain for their accent, their attitudes, their apparent stinginess, and their suspected loyalty to the godless Soviet Union. They filled the schools and the church we attended, ran most of the businesses in Mandan, and held political power in many small towns and in North Dakota as a whole. They owned the farms that stretched to the horizon beyond the edge of Mandan, and they populated many of the small towns in central and western North Dakota. In fact, in the forties and fifties, some of those towns—Streeter, Wishek, Ashley—were 100 percent German Russian. At home, in church, and even out in public, they spoke a dialect of German, which my mother called "low German" and they called "the language of the heart" and "God's language." They continued to observe cultural practices they had brought with them from their long sojourn in Russia. They munched on sunflower seeds, and the older women wore babushkas folded low over their foreheads. In St. Joseph's grade school all the cooks were German Russian, stocky, black-haired women who frequently cooked dishes straight from the Russian steppes. I couldn't swallow the borscht, thick, red, and warm as blood. Even today, in the cafes in Mandan, you can order up *fleischkuechle* and *knoephla* soup.

Many German Russians were my dad's friends, people who came to our store every week for decades, bought vegetables or fruit, and stayed to talk politics. But in the plainest terms, my father despised them as a group. He considered them ignorant, clannish, set in their ways, tight with their money, and hard on their women. (He told us that one man made his wife hitchhike to the hospital when she was in labor.) As we went off to high school and then college, one longtime customer asked my dad why he was bothering to educate all those girls.

Judy was only a few days into first grade when she noticed that she and her classmates didn't talk the same brand of English. She was unhappy about it and told my dad, "I sound different from the other kids." His swift and adamant reply was, "You're damn right you do, and you can be proud of it." Rather than trying to fit in with the German Russian majority, Dad urged us to hold ourselves apart from them and, of course, above them.

Dad didn't have to be able to see the German Russians to know who they were. Their strongly accented English is so distinctive that I'd recognize it anywhere. Lawrence Welk, who grew up and learned to play his accordion in Strasburg, a farming town southeast of Mandan, became the most famous German Russian in the United States. Every Saturday night on national television, Lawrence and his troupe of musicians and dancers entertained a big part of the country with his "champagne music," his lightning fingers playing the accordion, and his light feet showing the whole country how to dance a mean polka, schottische, or old-time waltz. He didn't try to sound like a network newscaster. I don't think he could've made his voice sound generic and urbane even if he'd wanted to. Instead, he put his German Russian accent out there for the whole country to hear and imitate as he set the beat: "A-one and a-two and a-three." Like the rest of the country we watched good old Lawrence every Saturday night and sang and danced along. Though my sisters and brother and I silently rejected most of my dad's ethnic prejudices, and Judy got into harsh Sunday-morning battles with him about black people and segregation, I don't remember any of us challenging his disdain for German Russians.

When I came to St. Benedict's Monastery in 1964, I soon discovered that I wasn't the only person from Mandan. Because Benedictine sisters had taught, nursed, and administered hospitals around Mandan and Bismarck since the 1870s, young North Dakota women interested in joining a religious order often went to St. Joseph, influenced by the women they'd known most of their lives. Some of these young women became homemakers and cooks, famous for noodles and pastries. But for fifteen hundred years Benedictines have educated women. So, like the Germans, Irish, and Poles, the German Russians who entered St. Benedict's Monastery became musicians, theologians, English teachers, school principals, nurses, hospital administrators. I'm ashamed to say that I was surprised to see their intelligence and varied gifts. How could these smart, talented women be the "dumb Russians" of my childhood? Only in pondering the question of prejudice's deep roots did I think to ask who the German Russians were and are, apart from my dad's opinions and my threadbare memories. I've learned that the "infinity of traces" their history left on them is remarkably similar to the traces history left on the Irish and should have made these two groups kin. But we didn't know their history. Many of them didn't know it. Like the Irish, the German Russians were busy forgetting what they could and hiding what they couldn't forget. Here is a small part of that buried history.

Between 1764 and 1823, thousands of Germans emigrated to Russia at the urging of Catherine the Great. Russia's vast steppes needed farmers, and the emigrants wanted to escape Germany's religious strife, high taxation, and the draft. By 1898 almost 2 million colonists lived in three thousand German-speaking villages. Catherine and succeeding Russian rulers granted them free land, freedom from conscription, and a degree of self-determination. They could continue to speak German and live and worship as they had in Germany. Their hard work and skill as farmers turned vast open lands into "a paradise on the steppe," where wheat, fruit, and vegetables flourished, and red cattle grazed.

The paradise lasted until the last decades of the nineteenth century, when Czar Nicholas demanded that the Germans become real Russians, speaking the Russian language and surrendering their sons to the army. The Germans were afraid that they would soon lose the freedom to worship as they wished. Between 1872 and 1914, three hundred thousand Germans uprooted their families and made the terrifying sea crossing to the United States and Canada. Those who stayed behind were all but wiped out by the famines that followed the 1917 Bolshevik revolution and the brutality of the Stalinist years. The government seized farms and destroyed churches. Between 1914 and 1945 more than a million Germans died from war or famine or from the deprivations of Siberian forced labor camps. Though individuals survived, the distinctive German community was destroyed.

The hundreds of thousands who came to the United States settled in villages delineated by religious affiliation. Though they often gave their towns German names—Strasbourg, New Leipzig—they also often built houses and impressive churches modeled on those they had left behind in Russia. Most of the North Dakota German Russians came from the area along the Black Sea, eventually settling over a hundred small towns in the state. As they had done in Russia, these brave, tenacious people suffered loneliness, unfamiliar farming conditions, and disease. In a few terrible weeks, diphtheria carried off all six children and a nephew in one family. Their short lives are marked by a line of crosses in the Zeeland cemetery. But the Germans from Russia had great powers of endurance. Besides, they were knowledgeable, adaptable farmers and ferocious workers, whose philosophy is captured in a couple of proverbs they carried with them from Russia: "Work makes life sweet," and "Prayer is of no use. What is needed is *misht*," or manure. They also brought with them from Russia the conviction that land, buildings, and livestock provided a more secure life than learning. They admired the successful farmer, not the teacher or scholar; the practical person, not the dreamer or storyteller.

Of course, these generalizations, too, are only partially accurate. The Germans from Russia are as complicated, surprising, and contradictory as any group of people. For instance, I never expected to learn from them about peace and nonviolence. In the United States, they sent their sons off to fight in one war after another and became fiercely patriotic, maybe to squelch doubts about their loyalty to the United States and their opposition to its enemies. Some of them were quick to condemn my brother and our family when he refused to fight in Vietnam. But historians describe them as gentle, peaceful people who left Germany and then Russia so that their sons wouldn't have to fight in wars waged by emperors and czars.

As I said, while they lived in Russia, the Germans kept to themselves to preserve their language, religion, and culture. But because they were surrounded by Russians and Ukrainians, they inevitably borrowed words, food, clothing styles, and mannerisms. After a century, they thought of Russia as their home and wept when they had to leave it. In the United States, they talked among themselves about "how it was back home in Russia," but until the 1970s many of them were quiet about their origins, ashamed of being German during World War II, and even more ashamed and fearful of being Russian during the McCarthy era and the Cold War. A 1999 Public Television special, *The Germans from Russia: Children of the Steppe, Children of the Prairie,* calls them "one of the most misunderstood ethnic groups" in the United States. Many of the million or so Germans from Russia scattered across the country don't know their own history, and, until recently, they had no way to learn it. The early settlers weren't writers or storytellers; their art was quilts and wrought-iron grave markers, which only the most discerning could interpret. Only in 1976 did the North Dakota State University at Fargo establish a heritage collection and begin to offer a course in their history and lead homeland tours.

As this brief history shows, the similarities between the Famine Irish in the United States and the Germans from Russia are so striking that one story could serve for both. Most obviously, both groups endured and somehow survived great sufferings: disease, famine, and religious, political, and cultural persecution. Both were people who loved their land and grieved when they had to leave it. The Irish held wakes for people fleeing the Great Hunger; the

Germans from Russia called emigration "half a death," and when the priest came to bless the travelers, he dressed in funeral black. Both the Irish and the Germans knew they were leaving land and family, never to return. Like the Irish, the Germans from Russia lived in small, closely knit communities and came together regularly to visit and to celebrate the feasts and rituals of their various religions: Catholic, Lutheran, Reformed, Mennonite.

I was amused and amazed to find small, homely likenesses I had never suspected. I thought the Irish had a monopoly on the derogatory nickname *potato eaters*, but historian Joseph Height reports that the German colonists grew such prodigious quantities of these lowly vegetables that the Russians called them "Katozchki," "potato eaters." Finally, like the Irish, the Germans from Russia loved music and dancing, and many homes in North Dakota had an accordion or a fiddle and someone who played it.

We didn't know about any of these similarities, but if we had, would it have made a difference in our attitudes? Or would we still have concentrated on the differences: the so-called Russian accent, the borscht, the indifference to education, and imaginary ties to the Soviet Union? Would these differences still have been an excuse to rank and judge?

I naively used to imagine that people who have suffered the diminishment of prejudice would recognize its narrowness and distortions and refuse to harbor it in themselves and bequeath it to their children. As I have shown in earlier chapters, both the Irish and the blind have faced prejudice from many quarters, right down through history. They know what it feels like to be the despised Other, their complex, unruly personhood reduced to one accidental feature of genetics or history. My father's words and actions and what I see around me in the United States have convinced me that the wounds prejudice has caused you and your people won't necessarily alert you to your own entrenched and unthinking judgments; nor will they always attune you to the sufferings your prejudgments cause or to the losses that come from writing off a whole group of people. Except for the potatoes, my description of the Irish and the Germans from Russia neatly fits most of the newly arrived immigrant groups looking for understanding and acceptance and often finding the opposite from those groups who have been in the United States a few generations longer.

Several of the definitions of 'prejudice' suggest that it results from a lack of knowledge or experience. For instance, prejudice is "a judgment formed before due examination or consideration, a premature or hasty judgment." Knowledge, education, would then seem to be the best antidote to "bigotry, bias, intolerance, and discrimination," to "narrow-minded or hidebound" opinions. My education, like that of most children in the forties and fifties, was decidedly mixed. The Benedictine sisters at St. Joseph's grade school taught us that the children in our big red geography books who lived on Baffin Island, in the Congo, on the Malaya Peninsula, and on the Kirghiz Steppe were as much God's children as we were and equal to us in every way. But with no apparent sense of contradiction they also introduced us to Wopsy, a fledgling angel who taught whole classrooms full of Catholic grade school kids bad theology, imperialism, and the indelible lessons of race, blackness, and sin.

Our second-grade teacher read *Wopsy* and *Wopsy Again* aloud, and then we fought each other to be first to check the books out of the library. We loved this story of the little angel sent on his first assignment to guard a newborn baby in darkest Africa. The books are thrillingly filled with open fire pits, black panthers crouching on tree limbs, and missionary motorbikes that are forever breaking down. Wopsy is kept busy averting one disaster after another, especially in the days before his new charge is baptized. The baby has an African name, but Wopsy can't pronounce it, so he calls him Shiny. Asleep, Shiny is beautiful, but when he opens his eyes, what Wopsy sees in the soul of the black baby sets his wing tips trembling with horror. For he sees not just sin but original sin, the sinful essence of humanity, sin dark and dense enough to permeate the whole being of every child born on this fallen earth. Wopsy knows that if Shiny isn't baptized by the black-robed missionary on his motorbike, if he dies "in the state of original sin," he'll spend eternity in limbo. All the prayers of all the Catholic school children in the world could not ransom Shiny from limbo. We, like Wopsy, had to get busy before he died.

Under the influence of Wopsy and our teachers, we raided our piggy banks and begged our parents for money to buy pagan babies out of the darkness of sin. When a class had accumulated five dollars, we got a certificate, a picture, and the privilege of naming the African, Indian, or Chinese baby we'd rescued. (The babies were never white, and I never wondered why.) Some kids were rich and had their own babies to name; most of us had to settle for communal parentage, bringing a nickel or dime for the weekly collection. The walls of some classrooms were lined with certificates, though I don't know whether those students were unusually generous or well off or if their teachers were unusually good at shaking them down, evoking pity and a spirit of competition for souls. What did that five dollars pay for? I don't know. I learned very young that the sacraments weren't for sale, and I certainly didn't think that we were buying gas for the missionary's motorbike. The sisters called this practice "ransoming pagan babies," suggesting that the babies were being held captive by some kidnappers or enslaved, probably by the devil, possibly by their own benighted families and countries. With the exception of the witch doctor, Shiny's parents and tribe are good people but blinded to the true faith by an accident of birth. Africa, which I saw as a dark, undifferentiated mass, must have seemed to me not the state but the continent of original sin. Eventually, the blatant racism in this story dawned on our teachers, and it disappeared from St. Joseph's grade school, along with the practice of ransoming pagan babies. The lessons it taught were harder to root out because they reinforced common prejudices.

The sisters also taught us to fear godless Communism, the kind practiced in Russia, and they didn't say anything at all about the Japanese people surrounded by barbed wire in Fort Lincoln just south of Bismarck. They couldn't teach what they didn't know, and like my father and the rest of the United States, they had no access at all to the facts about the Japanese held in internment camps during and after World War II.

I heard the phrase *dirty Jap* so often from the adults around me that I thought it was one inseparable word. Accurate, compassionate information about Fort Lincoln and its unhappy prisoners didn't appear until 1985, in John Christgau's book, *Enemies: World War II Alien Internment,* still the only book about the camp. In 2003 the North Dakota Museum of Art and the United Tribes Technical College, which is now situated in the old Fort Lincoln internment camp, organized an exhibit titled *Snow Country Prison: Interned in North Dakota.* These two works reveal for the first time what happened behind the " 'curtain of censorship,' which had been drawn over Fort Lincoln." Between 1941 and 1946 four thousand Germans and Japanese were held at Fort Lincoln. They weren't prisoners of war but rather United States citizens or legal aliens who were deemed security risks. The men who guarded them signed an oath swearing that they would never talk or write about what happened in the camps. Because my dad's cousin, Jim

Maloney, was a guard at the camp, we knew of its existence. In fact, we stayed there during one of the yearly spring floods. But many people in Mandan and Bismarck didn't even know that Fort Lincoln, a military post, had been turned into one of eight internment centers across the county to detain "enemy aliens" and that after the bombing of Pearl Harbor, many of those enemies were Japanese. When the camp was about to be closed in 1946, the press was invited in for the first and last time. The *Morton County News* described "Nazis and Sun Worshipers too dangerous to be loose in a world at war." Obviously, this description did nothing to dispel anti-Japanese "bigotry, bias, intolerance, or discrimination" based on ignorance.

With the help of the Freedom of Information Act of 1966, Christgau read hundreds of FBI files and interviewed both former inmates and guards, some of them now willing to talk. He paints a varied and sympathetic picture. While some of the Japanese internees were openly hostile to the United States, others wanted to enlist on the United States side (they were refused). Many of the eighteen hundred Japanese men housed in Fort Lincoln during those five years were devoted family men who had been forced to leave parents, wives, and children in camps in California and New Mexico. All they wanted was to be reunited with them, but they didn't know how to make that happen. Should they renounce their United States citizenship and agree to go back to Japan, or should they renounce Japan and pledge allegiance to the United States?

One of these men, Itaru Ina, wrote a series of haiku which were part of the museum exhibit. He wrote:

> Autumn grief
> unbearable—
> I look at the children's photos.

BLIND PREJUDICE

In the field of white snow,
I starve for the love
of my own people.

The station is hot—
there's hatred
in the eyes looking at me.

The war has ended—
but I'm still in
the snow country prison.

If the people of North Dakota had read his bitter, lonely words in 1945, we might have been moved to pity and outrage. But this knowledge, this priceless education, came sixty years too late to prevent prejudice and the injustice that always follows from it.

But knowledge doesn't always erase prejudice, any more than fellow suffering does. For there is body memory, long training, old fears and humiliations at the hands of some or even one member of a group. I've heard many people invoke the authority of experience to justify their prejudices. I grew up hearing claims such as these: "You wouldn't like Negroes if you'd been in the army and had to live with them." Or, from my high school friend, "You wouldn't like Negroes if you lived in St. Louis. We had a black maid, and she stole from us." But if personal experience is treacherous ground for judgment, inherited experience is even more so. My dad learned from his Irish parents, grandparents, and neighbors to hate the English, even though they were far away from that remembered oppression, and no English person ever set foot in Leaf Valley, Minnesota. These entanglements can overwhelm in an instant even the most capacious knowledge and the most generous impulses. Whether we mean well or ill, we're sometimes caught in prejudice's old web.

One Easter Sunday when I was about ten, our whole family marched up the front steps of St. Joseph's Catholic Church. As always on Sunday, my sisters and I were clean and starched and curled, with new dresses our mom had sewed for us and new hats perched on our heads. A little Indian boy was standing all alone on the church steps, his back pressed against the black iron railing. He was wearing a white shirt and black pants, both too big for him, and outsized men's dress shoes; his delicate brown hands were washed but with dirt ground into the creases. He was crying, and the tears made dirty streaks on his face. Two of my sisters and I saw him at the same moment, and I saw my own tears in their eyes. Without a word to each other, we all took the money we'd earned somehow and had brought for the collection plate and tried to put it in his hand. Then we tried to lead him into church with us. He didn't speak or even look up. He just stood there, resisting, with silent tears running over high brown cheek bones and past the downturned corners of his mouth. Maybe my sisters and I were being sentimental or patronizing, but I don't think so. We wanted him to join us in the long pew we filled end to end. He was our brother, and we wanted him to be part of our family. But all these years, I've wondered what the boy thought and felt. Were we three more white people trying to force pity and charity on him? Did our clean whiteness, our apparent closeness as a family, make him feel even more sharply how alone and different he was? Through that long, jubilant, miserable Easter Mass, I felt what I now know: no words or actions of ours could have erased several centuries of prejudice against this boy and his people; nothing could have made our loving gesture anything but an insult.

Sometimes the entangling web is outside us; sometimes it's inside; sometimes it's both. One day when I was in college and working a summer job in Mandan, I went into Woolworth's Dime Store for lunch. It was 1958 or 1959, just before black students began staging sit-ins at Woolworth's lunch counters all over the South and as far north as New York. The Civil Rights Act declaring racial segregation at lunch counters unlawful was still several years in the future. But I didn't need sit-ins or laws to know that segregation was wrong. On that summer day, I was about to sit down on an empty stool at the lunch counter when I saw that a black man was sitting on the next stool. I hesitated just long enough for him to see surprise and confusion on my face and for me to see his defensively raised shoulder and the cringing look in his eyes. The black man and I faced each other for a second, both of us heirs of three and a half centuries of prejudice, he reading fear and distaste in my hesitation—one more white girl afraid to sit next to a black man; I tripping over all I knew about racism and reverse racism, all I knew of history and especially that moment in history, and all I feared about entering the crowded country of loneliness. "I'll move," he said humbly and slid to the far end of the counter. I knew instantly that I'd done something terrible and that I couldn't undo it. Only a step as daring, clear, and defiant as those my dad had taken so often could have crossed the frozen distance separating my white self from his black self. Unlike my father, I couldn't take that step or unlock my tongue to say the simple, honest truth: "Don't move. I'd be glad to sit next to you."

Even when we're trying to resist it in and around us, prejudice blunders on at our borders and in our streets, schools, business places, churches, and government, new waves of it created by violence and fear. In the face of prejudice that spawns ever more violent children, children who have grown up armed with guns and grenades, it's tempting to renounce ethnicity, religion, gender, sexual orientation, all the distinctive marks that shackle us. It's tempting to shed our history and culture and just be humans in the company of other humans, free to accept or reject based on something other than someone else's old quarrels. Still, all around the world, forensic experts are "farming bones," to borrow the title of Edwidge Danticat's novel about the 1937 massacre of Haitians by the Dominican Republic. These experts are digging up mass graves in Guatemala, Bosnia, Sri Lanka, the Congo, Iraq, and a growing list of countries around the world to find the bodies of murdered and "disappeared" people, determine the cause of death, and, if possible, help bring the killers to justice. But does this farming bear the good fruit of justice and reconciliation or the poisoned fruit of another generation of ethnic, religious, gender, and tribal war? In the United States, we're fond of saying that we need to bury the dead so that we "can get on with our lives." My brother-in-law Roys Willenbring was an artillery forward observer in the Vietnam War. He wasn't surprised to learn about the torture at Abu Ghraib prison or Guantanamo or about the rape and murder of civilians in Iraq. He'd seen those things and worse and says that many Vietnam vets must be haunted by what they did in the chaos and moral confusion and ethnic hatred of that war. But if the Vietnam "conflict," as it is officially called, gets only a passing paragraph in most United States high school history textbooks, how are children to understand their haunted fathers, grandfathers, and uncles?

Unlike the blindfolded Lady Justice, my dad's blindness didn't make him an unbiased judge. He too was haunted by old hatreds that were given to him, and he cultivated some of his own. But this makes his many acts of resistance all the more remarkable to me. My sisters, brother, and I came out of our childhood confused but with questions rather than smug certainties. Prejudices from my childhood haunt me too, and I turn them up here not to stir up old quarrels or to justify or blame, but to acknowledge that all prejudices are blind and to lay them to rest.

SEVEN

Blind

Unable or unwilling to perceive or understand:
blind to a lover's faults.

Y FAMILY'S LIFE intersected many times with the
lives of the Mandan, Arikara, and Hidatsa Indians
who inhabited the Missouri River Valley for nine
hundred years, the last two hundred often disastrous for them.
The shelter of my memory holds story after story of moments
when our paths crossed, and we locked each other in the eye.
Until recently, I thought those encounters were purely personal
and considered myself unusually wide-eyed and accepting, even
a lover. Then, in doing research for another piece of writing,
I began to learn the history of these three tribes and to ask,
What happened? and why? and how? How can it be that the
slim luck my family enjoyed came at the cost of the Indians'
livelihood and culture?

GOING BLIND

To be specific, for fifty years I'd been blind to the fact that the Garrison Diversion Project, which ended the yearly flooding of our river-bottom land, displaced almost two thousand members of these tribes and destroyed their agricultural economy and their tribal culture. No white person, least of all me, asked the U.S. government what would be drowned under the waters of Lake Sakakawea, the wide, two-hundred-foot-deep reservoir created by the dam. The tragic history I've learned in the past couple of years is tied to the names, faces, and events that fill my memory. Those memories are an important prelude to the big impersonal story of the clash of cultures. Both the personal and the impersonal stories stun me with what I saw and even more with what I, my family, and my North Dakota neighbors didn't see. It has taken me sixty years to realize that many kinds of blindness are worse than the physical blindness that cast its shadow over our lives.

In a letter my dad wrote to my mother during the lonely weeks when she and his three little girls were visiting relatives in Minnesota, he said, "These Indians down here in the woods are half starving and I am afraid to leave the place alone too long." Poor as we were in November 1942, the Indians were poorer still, for my dad had a house and possessions to guard: a cow, a team of horses, the year's yield of potatoes. The Indians had much less.

An Indian woman named Bertha Blue Point worked for my parents, hoeing or weeding our enormous vegetable garden. She must have walked the two miles from Mandan, or, more precisely, from Dogtown, the dingy southside where she probably lived with her children in a tarpaper shack. I know nothing about her except her name. I don't remember her face or her voice. Maybe she never spoke. I do remember her sharp, rich smell and the sense I got from my parents that she was not as clean as we were. When Bertha drank from the old tin cup that hung from our outside pump–the one we all used–my mother scrubbed it before she'd let us drink from it again. I don't remember her scrubbing it for anyone else, not even Andy, the hired man, who chewed Copenhagen snuff.

I suspect that my parents were also afraid of her, thinking that Indians might steal children as well as potatoes and cows. I know my sisters and I were not afraid, as we stood in a semicircle and stared at her when she came in from the fields after a long day. She sat on an old trunk near the horse trough to drink cold water and pick cockleburrs from her clothes. Even in the hot summer sun she wore a long black dress and a blanket. She was a solid dark triangle, as stable as a boulder. It didn't look as if she could fall off the earth, so it didn't occur to me to be sorry for her. My family seemed to be in a more precarious position, hanging on to our mortgaged four acres and praying for good weather and fair prices. I didn't think to ask why Bertha Blue Point worked for us or why the Indians living in the woods near us weren't raising their own garden crops as we were.

Nor did I pity the carloads of Indian women who drove almost two hundred miles southeast from Mandaree on the Fort Berthold Reservation to Faulkner's Vegetable Market. They came every fall in the 1950s to buy vegetables for canning, loading their cars with generous bushels of cucumbers and tomatoes, buttercup and hubbard squash, peppers, corn, and onions. They bought the Indian way, or so my father said, paying in cash for one item at a time, peeling new bills from fat rolls of tens, twenties, and fifties. They never haggled over the prices as other customers did. They came to our store, I suspect, because my father remembered their names and never cheated them. He was kind and funny and liked to tease them.

I liked those women too, the way their dark faces creased into smiles as they exchanged bashful jokes with my dad and their almost silent laughter. I liked the complicated smell of their blankets and dark dresses that my nose breathed in and untangled: sweat, grease, wool, tobacco, wood smoke.

When I asked my dad where they got all that money, he told me what they told him, that the U.S. government bought their land from them to build the Garrison Dam. Blinded by those fistfuls of money in brown hands, I thought that was a fair deal. I never thought to ask what would happen when the ready cash from a one-time buyout ran out, how the Indians were now making a living, or how they felt about buying the vegetables they had raised for many generations on fertile table land. I don't know if any white person in North Dakota asked.

I did know, from years of experience, that we and other people living down river from Fort Berthold needed the Garrison Dam or thought we did. My family lived on the flood plain of the Heart River, a couple of miles east of Mandan. The Heart, a tributary of the Missouri, flooded almost every spring. The water usually crept toward our house, covering the garden and yard and filling the basement with brown water smelling of decay. Most years the ice thawed slowly, and we had ample time to put furniture up on blocks and move to a cheap motel in Mandan until the river receded and my parents could begin the nasty task of cleanup. Some years a member of the Army Corps of Engineers came out to tell my parents that they were going to dynamite the dike that held the water off our land. They had to do it, he said, to protect the city of Mandan. As he spoke, we heard the booming in the distance and knew we had to head to town. These weren't floods like the ones we've seen recently in Louisiana and Mississippi where tidal waves roused by hurricanes wash houses away. These floods moved slowly but inexorably out of the river's banks, across the fields, and into our basement. When dynamite blew a hole in the dike, the water came faster, and we sometimes drove to town at the last minute, with the water following us down the highway.

BLIND

Twice, in 1943 and 1952, the snow melted in a rush and ice gorged in the narrows, spilling millions of gallons of water onto the flats. In 1943 my parents had three little girls, aged four and under, and my mother was five months pregnant with the fourth. Dad had taken the cows and horses to higher ground, and when he got back, we were already marooned. He pulled on hip waders and walked to the high railroad track north of our house. Then he ran into town to get help for his wife and little girls waiting at home. I was almost three and remember the adventure of it: the four of us standing at our front door with the flood waters lapping at the sill, waiting to be rescued by men who came out from town on a railroad handcar. They rowed a boat to our house, helped us in, and rowed back to the railroad track. There we got on the wonderful car the men propelled by pumping a long lever back and forth.

I learned my father's side of the story later. Somehow, the messages got crossed, and when he got back to the house with his own boat, he found us gone. This man who had waited so long for the happiness of a family thought all of us had drowned. He was about to throw himself into the freezing flood water that would pull even a good swimmer under when he heard the shout, "Hey, Faulkner, we've got your wife and kids."

The Heart and the Missouri flooded again disastrously in 1952. This time the water poured into our basement and climbed the stairs to the high-water mark six feet up the walls on the main floor. It swallowed up my mother's creamy velvet wedding dress, the hide-a-bed where I slept between two of my sisters, my big doll Annie, her face washed away, our piggy banks, and the brilliant jars of food in the old gray wood fruit cupboard in the basement—jar after jar of ruby beets, emerald pickles, purple and orange jams thrown on the garbage heap.

Though the Heart still sometimes flooded the bottomlands, that was the last great flood in central North Dakota. By 1954, the

GOING BLIND

Garrison Diversion Project, begun in 1949, was well underway. My family and the many other white families living along the Heart and the Missouri would never again face that yearly terror. Few white people in North Dakota questioned the justice of the Army Corps of Engineers' decision or the fairness of the deal they offered the Indians. The history of the Mandans, Arikaras, and Hidatsas in North Dakota is the familiar story of disregard and betrayal, with no white people thinking to question until it was much too late to find answers. If we had asked the questions that occur to me now and listened to the answers, I doubt that the outcome would have changed, for our good luck blinded us to the cost.

I know something of the cost now, partly because I've done research, and partly because I feel, with rising terror, that we are all about to lose what the Three Affiliated Tribes of Fort Berthold, North Dakota, lost under the sluice of the water. As I said, I fell into this knowledge purely by accident. Browsing through a chronology of U.S. history, I stumbled on this little entry: "1949—Three Affiliated Tribes of the Berthold Reservation in North Dakota, displaced by the Garrison Dam and Reservoir Project, paid by the United States government $12,605,625 in land and damages."

For the first time in many years I remembered the dark women in my dad's store, their faces closed and somber until they smiled and the somberness broke into ripples and eddies of humor. But on all sides around those remembered faces rose the dark waters of my ignorance. I couldn't dredge up from memory what I'd never known. I could berate myself and my parents for knowing so little about them, except that most of their history and culture was lost before anyone thought it worth preserving.

The Pick-Sloan plan to dam the Missouri encompassed much more than the three small tribes in North Dakota. Besides the Garrison Dam, the plan proposed a system of a hundred and seven dams on the Missouri and its tributaries that create the vast Missouri Basin. This drainage area stretches from the Continental Divide in Yellowstone and Glacier Parks, through Montana and the Dakotas, along the Nebraska-Iowa and Kansas-Missouri borders, almost to St. Louis. The history of this project, which began as early as 1927, is a complicated story of political infighting between the Army Corps of Engineers, the Department of the Interior's Bureau of Reclamation, and a legislative plan that would have created the Missouri Valley Authority, a comprehensive program managed by a public corporation independent of powerful lobbies and vested career interests. While each of these wrangling bureaucracies proposed different methods of achieving their goals, the goals were similarly ambitious: flood control, which became politically urgent after the costly 1943 flood; improved navigation, to be achieved by deepening mud-choked channels; cheap hydroelectric power to light up far-flung ranches and farms; a reliable rather than a wildly capricious source of water for crop irrigation; fishing, boating, and swimming in the beautiful, clear reservoirs to be created by the dams, pleasures people living in dry states like North Dakota had rarely enjoyed; and finally the possibility of tourism for states outsiders rarely visited.

The Pick-Sloan Plan, a grudging compromise that eventually prevailed over the Missouri Valley Authority, was supposed to make life more predictable, prosperous, and comfortable for the white people living in an area encompassing half a million square miles in ten states. In the light of these bright promises, few noticed or cared that Indians lived in the "taking area" of many of the dams on land they'd been given by the U.S. government in earlier forced displacements. In *Dammed Indians: The Pick-Sloan Plan and the Missouri River Sioux, 1944–1980*, historian Michael Lawson writes, "The Pick-Sloan plan . . . caused more damage to Indian land than any other public works project in America." He details the suffering of dozens of native groups who lived along the Missouri and the other rivers dammed by this ambitious plan. While many tribes were disrupted by Pick-Sloan, Lawson says that "the most devastating effects suffered by a single reservation were experienced by the Three Affiliated Tribes (Mandan, Arikara, and Hidatsa) of the Fort Berthold reserve in North Dakota, whose tribal life was almost totally destroyed by the army's Garrison Dam." Sadly but predictably, the Garrison Dam was only the most recent of many betrayals, perpetrated blindly or with dazzlingly brutal vision against these creative, resourceful people.

When we were children, my family and friends and I sometimes picnicked, had birthday parties, and played cowboys and Indians at Fort Abraham Lincoln. This is a restored site on the bank of the Missouri River south of Mandan where several historical eras peacefully coexist in the present. A recent structure, built in 1989, is a faithful replica of the home where General George Custer and his wife, Libbie, lived. It's a spacious wood-frame house with wide porches looking out over the river bluffs and open to the constant wind, the scent of sage and sweet grass, and the songs of mead-owlarks. The antique furnishings include a fainting couch, a harp, and cages of zebra finches. Here Libbie Custer entertained the officers and their wives and visitors from back East; they danced and played parlor games like charades and Blind Man's Bluff. The army compound includes a barracks, a commissary, stables, and a mock graveyard whose headstones reveal the short, violent lives of frontier soldiers. On the nearby hills stand several block houses, two-story structures made of rough, vertical logs with rifle slots and lookout windows on the upper floor. Custer and his Seventh Cavalry were stationed at Fort Abraham Lincoln to protect the westward-moving railroad crews from Sioux attacks.

BLIND

Parts of this historical site were built in the 1930s by the Civilian Conservation Corps. The museum and gift shop have the CCC's unmistakable signature, both built of heavy, hewn stones and sturdy timbers that look as if they'll last forever. Like many plains museums, this one contains, side by side, exhibits of military artifacts; Victorian hats, gowns, and delicate shoes; and dioramas depicting seven hundred years of Indian civilization in the Missouri Valley, already a subject for anthropological study in the 1930s.

By the 1940s, when I first visited Fort Lincoln, the State Historical Society had constructed a replica of the On-a-Slant Village where the Mandan Indians had lived from 1575 to 1781. We played in the cool earth lodges, as rounded and smooth as pottery bowls. We tried out pine-bough sleeping mats along the walls and looked at the sky through the central smoke hole. When we got tired of being peaceful, the boys became marauding braves who caught the prettiest girls and tied them to the stake in the middle of the camp, threatening to burn them alive as we imagined the Indians had done. I grew up knowing Fort Lincoln, its smells, its feel, but it never once occurred to me to wonder why the Mandans left this beautiful place and what happened to them between 1781 and the 1940s and 1950s when they reappeared in our vegetable market.

My research unearthed a story that is familiar in its general outlines and shocking in its details. Until 1781, the Mandans were industrious, secure, hospitable people. Unlike the nomadic warrior tribes of Western lore, the Mandans lived in a permanent cluster of villages on both banks of the Missouri. At their most prosperous and healthy, more than fourteen thousand lived in nine villages. They were skillful hunters, farmers, diplomats, and traders, and while they defended themselves capably from attacks by the Lakota and other tribes, they didn't provoke battles. They didn't need to. The Missouri Valley was so fertile and the Mandan women such good farmers that after they'd stored away their winter supply of food, they still had a surplus of thousands of pounds of corn and other vegetables. The Mandan villages became a kind of trading bazaar that drew tribes and products from all four corners of the continent.

Why did the Mandans leave this hospitable place? The answer is familiar to every school child who's read about the diseases brought by white soldiers, fur traders, and settlers, against which the Indians had no immunity. The waves of epidemics in the eighteenth and nineteenth centuries were as devastating as the European plagues of the Middle Ages. In 1781 smallpox struck the Mandans. Within a few weeks, the disease had killed 11,000 of the tribe's 14,000 members. The survivors left their beautiful home, now piled high with the dead, and went north, joining forces with the Hidatsas at the mouth of the Knife River. The Hidatsas, too, had been almost wiped out by this epidemic, losing 70 percent of their 5,500 members. These small bands were just beginning to rebuild their lives when smallpox struck again in 1837. This time 1,500 of the 2,500 Hidatsa men, women, and children died. That same epidemic struck the Mandans. Out of 1,600, 125 survived. These are only numbers, not stories of a grief too vast to imagine. Were the survivors children or parents or old people? How could 100 people bury and mourn more than 1,400 dead? Of the survivors, only one name remains: Four Bears, whose face was so marred by smallpox, so the story goes, that even the timber wolf looked away in pity.

The second familiar story is of promises made and broken and the systematic attack on communal tribal ownership and governance. For over a hundred years, the three tribes were friendly with white traders and explorers. Lewis and Clark's Corps of Discovery arrived at the Knife River settlement of the Mandan and Hidatsas in 1804 just as a harsh winter set in. The Indians welcomed the explorers into their lodges and shared their store of winter food, probably saving them from starving or freezing to death. George Catlin, the eastern artist who lived with many western Indian tribes, painted at a furious speed to preserve on canvas peoples and civilizations he saw as threatened by disease or the "sword of civilizing devastation." Catlin especially liked and admired the Mandans and Hidatsas, whose rituals and games alternately horrified and delighted him. In one of his letters back home, he wrote: "A better, more honest, hospitable and kind people, as a community, are not to be found in the world. No set of men that ever I associated with have better hearts than the Mandans, and none are quicker to embrace and welcome a white man than they are . . and no man in any country will keep his word and guard his honour more closely." The Arikara also served as scouts for Custer's army against their traditional enemies, the Lakota or Sioux. This long friendship made later betrayals all the more bitter.

In 1851, the Hidatsa and Mandans moved to a reservation near Fort Berthold, two hundred miles northwest of Mandan; the Arikara joined them in 1862, on 12.5 million acres of river bottom, benchland, and upland prairie. The Treaty of Fort Laramie guaranteed that this land would belong to the three tribes "for as long as the waters flow." That promise lasted until 1887. For those twenty-five years, the three tribes owned the land communally and lived in several villages. The main one, where the tribal center was situated, was Like-a-Fishhook, a large village that bent to fit the curve of the Missouri. Having lived along the Missouri for almost eight hundred years, these people knew her moods and caprices, her life-giving brown waters, and the rich possibilities of the soil deposited yearly along her banks. As early as the seventeenth century, the Mandans had diverted the Missouri to irrigate corn fields. They were skilled farmers, who had taught agriculture to other upper

Missouri tribes. Even so, the dry, harsh, wind-scoured climate of northwest North Dakota must have posed a challenge. The temperature ranged from 56 degrees below in the winter to 112 degrees above in the summer; average frosts came as late as May 28 and as early as September 14, granting a scant 109 frost-free days with an average of fourteen inches of precipitation annually. "They can give North Dakota back to the Indians!" my mother used to say, not out of generosity but out of frustration at the almost biblical scourges that swept across northern and central North Dakota year after year. How was an uprooted Minnesota woman, used to lush, rainy summers and rich soil, supposed to feed her family when the garden was regularly drowned out, dried out, hailed out, or frozen out? How was she to grow flowers, keep the house clean, keep her mind intact when the wind never stopped blowing?

The women of the three tribes at Fort Berthold found a way to do all those things. In communal gardens, they grew twelve varieties of corn, winter squash, pole beans, small green melons, turnips, sunflowers, and pumpkins. They also harvested seventy species of wild plants, among them chokecherries, June berries, buffalo berries, wild currants, wild grapes, wild strawberries, and wild plum, blooming white and fragrant in the brief spring and producing tart fruit to dry. They used cattail down to insulate baby cradles, and the men hunted more than twenty-five species of wild game, most of them now rare or extinct in this area. In those few years, the tribes again prospered and grew.

Maybe it was this ability to survive on supposedly untillable land that led the U.S. government to take a second look at this and many other Indian land holdings. At this late date, it's probably impossible to sort out the mix of motives that led to the Dawes Severalty Act of 1887: greed for land on the part of farmers and speculators, a blind faith in the bracing virtues of individual ownership, a concern for the immortal souls of Indians who were still practicing the "old religion," and the perverse conviction that Indians would be productive U.S. citizens only when they were stripped of their traditional leaders, their culture and religion, and their economic independence. As Lawson says, agents of the Indian Bureau tried to make them "economically dependent on the government dole."

While the motives may be hidden in the thickets of the past, the effects of the Dawes Act on the Fort Berthold Tribes are all too visible. This act broke up communal ownership by doling out land in plots of 160 acres to the head of a household and 40 or 60 acres to dependent members. Any remaining land was opened up to white homesteaders. As Lawson says, "Humanitarians had long demanded that each Indian be given a farm, where the civilizing qualities supposedly inherent in tilling the soil could be readily absorbed." The administrators of the Dawes Act apparently ignored the fact that the Fort Berthold tribes had been tilling the soil for hundreds of years; they also ignored the nature of the land along the river. Years later, just as the waters of Lake Sakakawea were about to sweep over it, anthropologists took a good look at the flood plain and described it as "sandy alluvial loam, rich and friable, . . . ideal for hoe cultivation after the brush cover is removed." The Three Affiliated Tribes knew all this, growing crops and using methods in harmony with their land. Apparently they weren't the kind of farmers the Indian Bureau had in mind. Agents urged the tribes to abandon their gardens and become market farmers, growing wheat and small grains, which obviously require expensive reapers and threshers rather than hoes. The Dawes Act didn't specify inheritance, so when a male owner died, the land was divided among his heirs, breaking an ancient cultural pattern. Before this decree, the garden plots had been owned by the women and passed down in the matrilineal line. By 1910, each family at Fort Berthold owned a tiny square on the Missouri.

Belonging to a Benedictine monastery that follows a fifteen-hundred-year-old rule, I understand a little about the common life and the valuing of women and their work. Because of my mother, I also understand inheritance in the matrilineal line, not of property but of ways of working. My hands learned from hers how to mix, roll, and crimp a perfect pie crust, how to pack little cucumbers into the shoulders of Kerr jars for pickling, how to listen for the ping of sealed jars, how to pick a mess of lamb's quarters for supper. By the time I was seven, I could hoe and weed and rarely mistook a vegetable for a weed.

Even though I understand community and the passing on of essential skills from hand to hand, I don't pretend to know what this disruption meant for the people of the Affiliated Tribes. Still, I hear the grief in Buffalo Bird Woman's words, recorded and translated in 1917 by Gilbert L. Wilson: "I am an old woman now. The buffaloes and black-tail deer are gone, and our Indian ways are almost gone. Sometimes I find it hard to believe that I ever lived them. . . . Often in summer I rise at daybreak and steal out to the cornfield; and as I hoe the corn I sing to it, as we did when I was young. No one cares for our corn songs now." Our mother, a true monotone, didn't sing to her plants. But she had what I think of as her work song, a steady, cheerful "tnk, tnk" made by clicking her tongue against the roof of her mouth. That's the song she sang as she worked her way down the long rows of peas, cucumbers, and tomatoes. During her sixty years as a gardener, she learned pretty much all there is to know about planting, growing, and harvesting crops. After my dad died in 1965, Mom had to make a living for herself and Mona, her youngest daughter, who was still in grade school. Over the next twenty-eight years she built

Faulkner's Market into a busy seed and plant store. Every spring thousands of people came from as far away as the Montana border to buy their seeds and listen to Mom's free gardening advice. She handed on her plant lore to my sister Elaine, who took over the market in 1993 after Mom died, and who now presides, answering a steady stream of questions, sometimes using Mom's very words. The women and men of Fort Berthold never got to hand on to children and grandchildren their knowledge of gardening, farming, hunting, and ranching. That knowledge, like so much essential tribal and religious knowledge, was cut off abruptly and eternally.

Buffalo Bird Woman said: "Sometimes at evening I sit, looking out at the big Missouri. The sun sets, and dusk steals over the water. In the shadows I seem again to see our Indian village, with smoke curling upward from the earth lodges; and in the river's roar I hear the yells of the warriors, the laughter of little children as of old. It is but an old woman's dream. Again I see but shadows and hear only the roar of the river, and tears come into my eyes. Our Indian life, I know, is gone forever."

Hearing this elegy for a lost way of life, it's hard to imagine that the Garrison Dam could further damage these tribes, but it did. After 1887 the Three Affiliated Tribes picked up the thread of their tribal life again. Evidence of their resilience and tenacity comes mainly from the reports of anthropologists and paleontologists, and not, until recently, from the Indians themselves.

In 1950, four groups embarked on the Inter-Agency Archaeological Salvage Program, coordinated by the Smithsonian Institution and the National Park Service. At Fort Berthold, as in all the reservoir areas, archaeologists, paleontologists, and historians excavated dozens of sites, publishing their findings in the *River Basin Survey Papers*. Their reports are respectful, scholarly, and objective, making no judgments about the rightness or wrongness of what the federal government was doing to the Indians. The scholars often took refuge in the passive voice, as if no person or agency were responsible for the decision to divide and flood Indian land, or as if the water itself were to blame. For instance, in his 1955 report on "small sites on and about Fort Berthold Indian Reservation, Garrison Reservoir, North Dakota," George Metcalf wrote: "Much more evidence from such sites will be required before the culture or cultures represented can be adequately described and properly placed in the Plains cultural sequence. Unfortunately, such data may never be forthcoming, for even as these lines are being written the rising waters of the Garrison Reservoir are rapidly placing most of the sites beyond the reach of the archaeologist."

Metcalf adds this carefully detached comment: "Such information as remains in the ground is now lost forever beneath the waters of the Garrison Reservoir." I hear in his voice regret for the loss of knowledge and the disruption of scholarly inquiry but no hint that he mourns the loss of a way of life for three tribes who had faced extinction many times but who had, until then, adapted and survived. Whether the scholars saw that loss or were blinded by their preconceptions I don't know. They never say.

Besides recording garden and farm crops, and such bric-a-brac as "Sensation Play Tobacco," "portion of a plate made in England," and "toothpaste jar lid," the archeologists also described existing structures, such as the last Arikara earthlodge built in 1908. An early surveyor surmised that this earthlodge showed that the Arikara had "reverted to their early religion." Its entrance faced the rising sun, but this lodge seems to me to indicate an ending rather than a hopeful beginning: even for the tribes, ceremonies and ceremonial spaces were artifacts constructed to teach the young about a vanishing way of life. Whatever it represented of the past or the present, by the time the archaeologists had published their reports, the lodge was decomposing under the waters of Lake Sakakawea.

BLIND

Again from the *River Basin Survey Papers* comes the distant voice that refuses to acknowledge choice or responsibility: "Right-of-way for the Garrison Reservoir necessitated the acquisition by the Federal Government of over 150,000 acres of Indian land, and the filling of the reservoir will split the reservation into five residual segments." Those are the facts, but let me make them more precise: without consulting the three tribes, the Army Corps of Engineers designed a reservoir that would cover 152,360 acres of bottomland, 94 percent of the tribes' agricultural land. More than three hundred families—80 percent of the tribal population—would need to move. The water would drown seven Indian towns—Independence, Lucky Mound, Charging Eagle, Shell Creek, Red Butte, Beaver Creek, and Elbowoods—and in those towns, tribal headquarters, a hospital, and many religious and burial sites. "The Flood that Stayed Forever," or simply "The Flood," as the Indians called it, would eventually cover floodplain timber (which the Corps didn't let the Indians cut before inundation), natural habitat for game animals, winter cover for deer and livestock, wild plant foods, and whatever minerals might have been discovered on the land. As the *Basin Survey Papers* say, the flooding divided Indian land into five small parcels, each surrounded by a wide, deep moat, moving the Indians so far apart that they couldn't come together to celebrate, dance, or hold rituals; they couldn't work together or help each other out. In exchange for their bottomland, the Corps offered them high, arid range land, from which no soil samples had been taken. As tribal chair Martin Cross told the Senate Select Committee on Indian Affairs in 1945, the land was "fit for rattlesnakes and horned toads." The Indians protested every part of the Corps' plan. An elder named James Driver, one of hundreds of Indians who came to a meeting in Elbowoods called by Colonel Pick, expressed a common sentiment: "The land beneath our feet is the dearest thing in the world to us, and I am here to tell you that we are going to stay here. We refuse to be flooded." Understanding neither the Indians' spiritual connection to their land nor their sense of betrayal by a government they had trusted, Pick and his aides left the meeting in a fit of anger. In the end all protests were futile. In 1947 the Corps gave the tribes a take-it-or-leave-it offer: Accept $33 an acre ($2600 for someone who owned 60 acres; $5280 for 160, the largest parcels granted in 1887). The Indians went to court, negotiating for a fairer settlement. Two years later, in 1949, they received the government's final offer—$12.5 million, $9 million less than the land's assessed value. Newspapers across the country published a picture of the interior secretary signing the bill. Behind him, awkward in a pin-striped missionary-barrel suit, tribal chairman George Gillette weeps.

The "Taking Act" became law in 1949. Almost immediately, the Corps moved in with jacks and sledgehammers. People returned from shopping to find their houses and barns gone, hauled off on flatbed trucks by the Corps. Sometimes the dispossession happened with the owners inside. Late in 1954 the waters of Lake Sakakawea drowned the last of the Fort Berthold Indian villages. As historian Paul VanDevelder writes, "For the first time in nine hundred years, the winter moon would not rise on Mandan villages in the gooseberry woods of the Missouri River Valley."

These, too, are facts, accurate, harsh. If I, my family, and the other white people living in North Dakota's Missouri Basin had known them, what would we have said? That several white towns were also inundated by the reservoir (Sanish, VanHook, Roseglen); that the Indians, like everyone, had to change and adapt to progress; that North Dakota needed an attraction to draw tourists and their money to a state that everyone was always leaving; that there were still white farmers without electricity; that the Indian women were lucky to be free from the drudgery of growing their own food. And we who lived along the Missouri and her tributaries remembered well the floods of 1943 and 1952 and considered the dislocation of a few hundred Indian homes a small price to pay for our livelihood. We were so in love with our lives and, in those Cold War years, so in love with the United States, that we were blind to our government's tragic and repeated injustices.

My mother, most at home in her garden, would have understood that a brown woman's hands, used to the hoe and the plump heaviness of harvest-ready vegetables, but now holding only a wad of bills, would feel empty and useless. And I believe my father would have understood that men whose hard work and canny adaptability had supported their families would be humiliated by government handouts. But in 1954, my parents were struggling to support their own family. Mona, the seventh child, was a year old. Dad was fifty-nine, his health precarious and his vision almost gone. We couldn't afford to move, and we couldn't afford another disastrous flood. Even with knowledge and sympathy, my parents would have resorted to the familiar rationalizations. They wouldn't have asked the Indian people who came into our store what they had to give up in exchange for the fat rolls of money they held in brown hands.

VanDevelder writes that before the "Taking Act," life at Fort Berthold was economically and socially stable. Only 3 percent of the people received government assistance. During World War II, when many men from the reservation enlisted, women kept the farms profitable and the families intact. Most children came home to two-parent families, and the diseases and addictions that now plague the reservation were almost unknown, as were divorce and domestic abuse.

The Garrison Dam destroyed that stability almost overnight. Once the money they'd received for their land was gone, the people faced starvation. They found that Martin Cross had been right about the land "on the top"—rattlesnakes thrived there, but not crops or cattle. Still less could these communal people thrive on small parcels scattered across the broad and desolate plains. There were few jobs and growing racism in the white towns nearby. By 1982 unemployment stood at 85 percent, and four out of five children were malnourished. Carl Whitman, who was tribal chair during the worst of these years, names hostility, apathy, and self-destruction as the inevitable results when a group's whole way of life is taken from them. At Fort Berthold, he said, "They have all come to pass. I have witnessed these." Self-destruction is the most visible effect. Fort Berthold was quickly transformed into the all-too-familiar reservation stereotype, with broken families living in sheds or cars or on the street; alcoholism, drug addiction, and suicide rates climbing; and children dying of starvation, neglect, and exposure. Phyllis Cross, whose family was displaced and then dispersed across the country, says of those terrible years: "Our thinking failed us because suddenly . . . our social and physical landmarks, the framework of everything we were, was gone. Our identity derived from our villages. Those were destroyed. . . . What do you call your life as a community, as a people, when despair is the only emotion you can trust?"

To make matters worse, the federal government instigated a policy called "relocation," or, more honestly, "termination." The real goal was to end the treaty rights tribes claimed as sovereign nations within the nation of the United States and to eliminate tribes and reservations altogether. The euphemistically stated goal was "to liberate the Indian into mainstream society." To do that, the government bought Indians one-way bus tickets to big urban centers: Seattle, Los Angeles, Chicago, Denver, San Francisco. Within ten years, half of the Fort Berthold tribe had been "liberated," many of them disappearing into urban ghettoes.

BLIND

Shame and silence like that of the Famine Irish gripped the survivors of this disaster. It took several decades for members of the Three Affiliated Tribes to break that silence. Some went to college, becoming lawyers, engineers, and environmentalists, and returned to Fort Berthold to help rebuild the tribe one more time. In 1992, thanks to the skilled legal work of Indian lawyers (VanDevelder calls them "Coyote Warriors") and their allies, the United States government put $142 million in trust for the Three Tribes, as "just compensation" for the loss of their land and livelihood. The money is to be used for health, education, and economic growth. The tribes are now asking that thirty-six thousand acres of ancestral land bordering Lake Sakakawea be returned to them to be developed for recreation and tourism. Still, in spite of some economic development, such as the Four Bears Casino, and a community college, 35 percent of the people live below the poverty level, compared with 11 percent for North Dakota as a whole; unemployment on the reservation stands at 42 percent, ten times that of the rest of the state. The Garrison Dam, which promised prosperity to western North Dakota, has been an environmental disaster, and after years of drought, Lake Sakajawea is brown and sluggish. The reservation land will never be restored to its austere and fertile beauty.

In her introduction to the exhibit at the Strokestown Famine Museum in Ireland, former president Mary Robinson says that such exhibits "invite us to look steadily at a past we can neither share nor change." I think she's right, but I also think that attentive looking, apologies, and reparations don't mean a thing unless they contain what we Catholics used to call "a firm purpose of amendment"—the sincere promise that we won't commit this sin again. But as fresh water becomes scarcer and more precious, the damming of great rivers goes on around the world. And in the

United States, where most reservations are by design far from the lights of cities and suburbs, tribes are being offered millions of dollars and well-paying jobs if they will agree to store garbage, hazardous wastes, and spent nuclear fuel on their land. Some tribes have already accepted these offers from private waste-management companies and federal agencies.

At St. John's University and Monastery, in Collegeville, Minnesota, hundreds of people wander through a restored prairie. This and other restorations save the sights and smells of the disappearing prairie for the children of the twenty-first century and for the painters who set up their easels and capture this gray-green beauty in watercolors or oils. When I rub prairie sage between my fingers, its sharp, sweet smell releases the memories of my first eighteen years when my sisters, brother, and I wandered the hills near Mandan. Restoring a prairie is a long and labor-intensive project. Geneticists say that by midcentury, if we have so much as a shred of DNA, we'll even be able to clone extinct birds, plants, and mammals, so that some day pinky-tan passenger pigeons might again darken the sky. We might be able to undo our blind wantonness.

But there is no way to undo the destruction of the ancient Mandan, Hidatsa, and Arikara culture. The government is not going to blow up the Garrison Dam and drain the reservoir. And even if it did, you can't clone religion, drum rhythms, or dance steps, the souls of corn plants or Buffalo Bird Woman's corn song; still less can you clone the invisible threads that make a community and weave it together.

The college students who guide grade school kids through the earth lodges at Fort Lincoln tell them about a vanished people admirably attuned to their natural habitat. They tell about the epidemics that emptied this village and say that the last full-blooded Mandan Indian died in 1960. They encourage the young students to remember this culture that thrived for two hundred years right here, on these windy bluffs under the wide North Dakota sky.

The guides don't talk about the Garrison Dam or urge the students to visit Fort Berthold. I understand their silence. It's comfortable to relegate the Mandan, Arikara, and Hidatsa Indians to the reservation of memory, where they are romantically admired and safely distant from the present. But such romantic remembering is its own kind of blindness. The members of the Three Affiliated Tribes who have survived all the imperialistic decisions of the past are not museum artifacts. Nor are they the somehow substantial, somehow shadowy women and men I remember. They are people of the twenty-first century who, like all of us, carry their history with them. The next few decades will tell whether they and their land can recover and prosper.

EIGHT

Blind

Insensible, unaware, lacking intelligence and consciousness, narrow-minded with no openings or passages for light

M Y NEPHEW JEB ALSO has retinitis pigmentosa. At night he's "as blind as a horse's butt," as my sister Jeanne would say, and has severely restricted peripheral vision, which makes navigating dim, new, or crowded spaces very difficult. In the safety of his desk in a classroom or in front of a computer screen, his brilliant mind took over, but between classes in the chaos of crowded grade school and high school hallways, he was often lost. Sometimes he could follow the beacon of his friend's red hair or use his hands as a swimmer does to propel himself through the waves of careless humanity. But neither his intelligence nor these strategies fooled his classmates. They knew he saw a narrow slice of their world. One day one of them said to him, "If I had your eyes, I'd just kill myself and get it over with." Jeb's classmate was a messed-up junior high kid bent on meanness, but he was also expressing the deeply held and deeply hurtful perception of many sighted people that blindness is a fate worse than death. This perception is reinforced by the English language as the figurative uses listed above show, by Judeo-Christian symbolism, and by much of Western literature, all of which line up blindness, darkness, sin, and death on one side of the river of grace, and on the other, sight, light, goodness, and life. Blind and visually impaired people must wrestle with the distorted and constricting imagination that many, perhaps most, sighted people have of them and their lives. People who go blind gradually, after years of sight, have an especially hard time resisting this toxic imagination, which tells them with arrogant certainty what they feel, think, and are.

When I began this study of blindness, I read definitions like those above with dismay, realizing that one day they'd claim to describe me, too. While my father never consulted a dictionary or a thesaurus, these phrases and meanings were and are commonplace; they help me understand why he prayed so fervently for sight, refused to be reconciled to his blindness, and rejected the label *blind*, which would have described to others, including his children, not only his damaged retinas but also a defective mind, heart, will, and spirit. That tunnel vision he would not accept.

Nor will I, yet the intense gravity is hard to resist, for blindness slides into darkness, creating metaphors and figures of speech that soon lose their metaphorical tension and become statements about real people in the real world. "It's always darkest just before the dawn," my mother always said. Truisms like this one imply that blindness/darkness, whether physical, mental, or spiritual, is bad, or at least filled with unseen dangers, while sight/light is good. The familiar oppositions between blindness and sight, darkness and light, death and life, sin and redemption and their weighty connotations are burned into the imaginations of every U.S. inhabitant, every Jew and Christian, and perhaps every heir of Western civilization. Maybe looking at these oppositions is a way to challenge their power.

The references to light in Judeo-Christian scripture are far too numerous to cite. Light spills from the pages of these books, from the first chapter of Genesis, whose author describes God pushing back primeval darkness with the good light, through the psalms and the prophets, to the Gospels. The prophet Isaiah describes the coming Messianic kingdom as the coming of light:

> The people who walked in darkness
> have seen a great light;
> those who lived in a land of deep darkness—
> on them light has shined.

In John's gospel, Jesus says, "I am the light of the world; whoever follows me will never walk in darkness but will have the light of life." On the vigil of Easter, in our darkened church, we celebrate the fulfillment of that Messianic promise. The presider lights the tall Christ candle, singing three times, "Lumen Christi, Light of Christ." From that flame, the light spreads through the dark church as each worshiper lights the small candle of her neighbor. The light pushes the darkness back, making it a friendly, beautiful shelter.

In Catholic Church services, we sing dozens of songs that set up light and darkness as opposites:

> Christ, be our light!
> Shine in our hearts.
> Shine through the darkness.

We, like many other denominations, sing wholeheartedly and unquestioningly:

> Amazing grace, how sweet the sound
> That saves a wretch like me.
> I once was lost, but now am found,
> Was blind, but now I see.

It's true, of course, that blind people are often lost in space. One wrong turn, and even familiar terrain becomes strange and treacherous—an open stairway to tumble down, a busy street, a strange and suddenly hostile neighborhood. But the parallel lines of this song suggest that being blind, being lost, and being a sinner are similar wretched states that only God's grace can transform into their bright opposites.

Knowledge, whether before, after, or into an event, we call "sight": *foresight, hindsight, insight.* Ignorance is mental darkness. "Do you see?" we ask. We don't always trust our eyes. As the fox tells the Little Prince in Antoine de St. Exupéry's famous book, "Only with the heart does one see rightly. What is essential is invisible to the eye." Yet even that defense of the invisible is filled with seeing. Vision, which conventional wisdom believes requires only the cooperation of healthy eyes and light, is synonymous with the ability to see into the heart of reality and way beyond to where God dwells "in unapproachable light."

While no one now repeats out loud the old belief that blind people or their parents were being punished by God for sins or misdeeds, some contemporary books reinforce the ancient entanglement of blindness, darkness, and evil. One of the most recent is *Blindness,* written in 1995 by the Nobel-Prize-winning Portuguese author José Saramago. Saramago created a nameless modern city in a nameless

country where nameless people are suddenly afflicted with a plague
of blindness. It's a peculiar kind of blindness that descends not like
the night but like a milky whiteness in front of their eyes. When
the people in the city see how contagious blindness is, spreading
to the healthy "like the evil eye," they quarantine the blind in an
empty mental asylum to try to prevent the plague from spreading,
and then virtually abandon them, dropping off food rations at a
distance and promising to shoot anyone who tries to escape. Inside
the quarantine asylum most of the blind people quickly degenerate
into savagery. The self-appointed rulers are brutal, ignorant men
whose leader has a gun. They hoard the rationed food and then
sell it for sex, gang raping the women. Many of the blind men
urge the women to pay this price. Among the inmates, the only
person who can see is a doctor's wife, who pretends she's blind
so she can stay with her husband. Around her grows up a little
community whose members stick together, share what they have,
and look out for each other. But without her and her vision, the
others seem paralyzed by fear and lack of imagination. These blind
people have no ingenuity except the ingenuity of evil; they don't
sing or dance or pray, "for blindness is also this, to live in a world
where all hope is gone." The doctor, a kind ophthalmologist who
was one of the first to go blind, says fatalistically, "The charitable,
picturesque world of little blind orphans is finished, we are now in
the harsh, cruel, implacable kingdom of the blind." In this kingdom, no leaders will emerge because that would be "nothingness
trying to organize nothingness." The people outside the hospital
are no better than those inside; driven only by self-preservation,
they're willing to stoop very low to save their eyesight. For in this
city, blindness is a fate as bad as death or worse and leads many
to suicide. The blind people, led by the doctor's wife, eventually
escape and find a ruined city, where wandering bands of the blind

(for by now everyone is blind) loot stores and deserted homes for food. In the end the "white evil," like most plagues, disappears as mysteriously as it came.

Saramago must have had a reason to choose blindness as his plague of choice rather than deafness, let us say, quadriplegia or muteness, schizophrenia or AIDS, each of which has its own metaphorical charge. I believe that all the old perceptions and fears of blindness led him to choose this affliction. Think back to the list of synonyms at the beginning of this chapter. To be blind is to be *insensible, unaware, lacking intelligence and consciousness, narrow-minded with no openings or passages for light.* To that dismal litany, the thesaurus adds *reckless, possessed by blind fury; destitute of intellectual, moral, or spiritual light; insensible, unaware; inconsiderate, lacking affect.* Maybe those adjectives accurately describe the people of the modern world as Saramago sees us; they certainly characterize the suddenly blind people in this story. Readers will be quick to say that in this novel blindness is only a symbol and that these are not real, live blind people. But a curious slippage often happens between symbol and the thing symbolized. The object or person used as a symbol is endowed in reality with the qualities of the thing symbolized, especially if the symbol is repeated so often that it begins to seem like a natural correspondence. In addition, Saramago includes in his cast of characters one man whose blindness is not metaphorical but literal. He was blind before the plague struck and brings his Braille writer to the asylum when he's swept up with the hordes of the suddenly blind. Instead of being a leader who teaches the others the skills he has obviously learned, he becomes the accountant for the armed men who have seized control, using his Braille writer to keep track of food doled out and sexual favors received. Saramago's novel is a terrifying allegory, but it does no favors for blind people. Rather, it is one more blind hedge, hiding them from sight in their full and beautiful humanity.

BLIND

Most sighted people would never say out loud the terrible senti-
ments Saramago expresses in *Blindness,* nor would they repeat the
cruelty of Jeb's classmate. Still, many failures of imagination persist,
creating misunderstanding and needless pain. One of the women
Stephen Kuusisto meets at Guiding Eyes for the Blind says that
real sighted people, like Saramago's fictional ones, try to get out
of the way of real blind people: "Yeah, well, they're afraid you'll
bump them, and then they'll be blind too—everyone knows that
blindness is like a game of freeze tag!" I can think of only one
way to challenge this intense imagination of despair, and that is
to ask visually impaired and blind people what their inner worlds
are like and how they relate to the outer world. The second step
is to listen to their varied, unruly, often contradictory answers that
shift from person to person and from day to day and even from
moment to moment.

Many people imagine that sight and blindness are polar opposites and the only possible alternatives for the human eye. In
reality, as people with RP, macular degeneration, and a host of
other conditions will tell you, there's a whole range of possibilities
between these poles. That ambiguity is hard to handle for many
sighted people, who want their world black or white, blind or
sighted, but not confusingly and unreliably gray or multicolored.
My nephew Jeb says:

> Most sources of pain for me . . . arise from two forms of mis-
> understanding. The first kind stems from those who think we
> see much worse than we do. These people tell us to buy canes
> and learn Braille. Then there is the opposite—those who see
> us as sighted. We don't need canes and we can read a book,
> so why don't we drive? They think we must be faking the
> other times, the times when we can't see the math problem
> on the black board or the empty seat on a dark bus or the

hand stretched out in greeting. I've been chewed out by lots of teachers, bus drivers, and many, many fellow students who somehow can't detect my vision problems. This may be the worse of the two sources of confusion.

My nephew Chad, who also has RP, sometimes uses a cane at night to walk from his work to the bus stop. Imagine the confusion and indignation of the other riders when he gets on the bus, folds up his cane, and starts to read his newspaper. No doubt some consider him a phony or a freeloader using his white cane to claim a handicapped seat on a crowded bus.

Another misconception about blind people, based upon faulty imagination, is that they, like blindness, are monochromatic in their feelings, convictions, fears, and dreams. Research and my memory of my dad have taught me the opposite. As with any group of people who have one quality in common, the differences among them are far too numerous to list, but understanding a couple of striking contrasts in convictions has helped me.

Some blind people, usually those who've been blind from birth or from a very early age, are so at home in the world that they don't want or need special accommodations. They find unnecessary, unhelpful, and demeaning such innovations as talking traffic lights that tell everyone when it's safe to cross the street. They argue that real empowerment comes not from having all obstacles removed—an unrealistic expectation—but rather from teaching blind people to meet them with poise, ingenuity, and confidence. Others, often those who lost their vision later in life, worked hard for the passage of the Americans with Disabilities Act and now push for adaptations in public places and full access to jobs. Some people use canes; some have guide dogs; some use neither. Some learn Braille, while others depend on talking books, reading machines, and computers. Each of these adaptations has its champions. Some blind people say they can do anything they set their minds to; others name many real, intractable limitations. Some put their hope, energy, and resources into finding cures so that eventually RP or macular degeneration will not be a sure prelude to blindness, any more than cataracts are now, at least in developed countries. Others urge everyone to stop thinking about blindness and other physical and mental disabilities as tragic imperfections that need to be cured, no matter the price.

Another important difference among blind people, one on which many other differences hinge, has to do with imagination itself, the creation, representation, and recreation of images in the mind. While it's true that the very word *image* commonly means "visual representation," even many people with 20/20 vision don't think primarily in pictures, turning instead to words, music, numbers, formulas, shapes, textures, and configurations of space. Oliver Sacks, who calls himself a neuroanthropologist and is as interested as I am in the wild, mysterious gift of imagination, describes both sighted and blind mathematicians, biologists, and surgeons whose imaginations are primarily spatial and tactile, and some who can't call up any visual images at all.

Like many activities, from walking and eating to finding the restroom in a dim bar, exercising the imagination is one that blind and visually impaired people have to pay attention to in ways that sighted people do not. For a long time I've wondered what happens to the inner world, the imagination, of a visually orientated person like my dad, when he can't see any longer. Without new images to feed his imagination, did his wide inner world shrink and collapse in on itself, getting tiny and claustrophobic? I think this question is bigger than the narrowness or spaciousness of my dad's mind, though I will begin there. For me, this question opens up an array of additional questions that may be important to us as humans, bodily creatures who learn though our senses.

It's true that my dad had honed his other senses, reveling in music and movement. Even in heavy work shoes, he was light-footed and graceful, a dancer. While most of us have to remind ourselves to use senses other than sight, he learned and judged by touch. Because his failing sight demanded that he hold objects very close to see them at all, he often gained knowledge from his more immediate senses. He picked things up, hefted them, felt their size and texture, let his fingers distinguish between crabgrass and the feathery tops of carrots or smooth beet greens. Once when we were very young my two sisters and I were playing in the cow pasture near our house. We found in the grass a golden-brown coil, silky and pleasant to the touch. We trooped over to where our dad was working in the garden, carrying our sinuous treasure. "Daddy, we found a silky rope!" He took it and held it an inch from his better eye. But it was his hands that told him our silky rope was a garter snake, alive and cool, that had been sleeping in the pasture. He flung it away, a shining arc in the sun.

Hearing, touch, smell, and taste certainly gave him ways to know his world. Still, stories I remember and those my sisters have told me make me think that Dad's blindness sometimes locked his imagination in the past or led him down blind alleys. They also make me think that he'd always been an intensely visual person, one who habitually paid attention and remembered what he had seen. After I graduated from college in Minnesota, my parents decided to stop at my dad's home farm on the way back to Mandan. The only problem was that the farm was gone. Still, after forty years, my dad directed Mom, the direction-blind driver, unerringly to the spot, now marked only by an artesian well and an old pump.

BLIND

The visual images he carried in his mind were those he formed in the first forty years of his life: the road to his childhood home, clothes, hairstyles, houses, even colors. The world, naturally, left those images in the dust. After many years of living in our small house, my parents finally had enough money to add a few rooms, put in indoor plumbing, and modernize the kitchen. My mom had been poring over *Good Housekeeping* magazines and drawing house plans with Judy for twenty-five years. She knew what she wanted. One day, well into the remodeling, she said she'd like to paint the new kitchen aqua. My dad didn't say anything, but later he asked Coreen, one of the two kids still at home, just what aqua looks like. Her description—a sort of blue-green—probably didn't conjure up an image in his mind to counter the white or yellow or cream kitchens he remembered. I don't think he ever saw, even in imagination, my mother's pride and joy, her new aqua kitchen.

Dad remembered and sang dozens of songs, some new, most old. One was called "Among My Souvenirs," and he crooned it to our mom in a voice as rich as barley broth. He sang it as a love song, with a little half-smile on his face. Even though it's a song about lost love, it didn't seem sad then; or maybe it seemed to be that delicious kind of sadness you want to feel so you can sing about it, too:

> There's nothing left for me
> Of days that used to be
> They're just a memory
> Among my souvenirs.
>
> Some letters sad and blue
> A photograph or two
> I see a rose from you
> Among my souvenirs.

GOING BLIND

A few more tokens rest
Within my treasure chest
And, though they do their best
To give me consolation,

I count them all apart
And, as the teardrops start,
I find a broken heart
Among my souvenirs.

Now, when I read the words, they seem to describe visual images and their accompanying feelings trapped in the past.

It's too late to ask my dad whether his imaginative world stagnated or flourished, but my reading has presented me with several fascinating possibilities, consciously chosen and recorded by people who went blind after their imaginative worlds were well formed. On one side is John Hull, whose journal, *Touching the Rock: An Experience of Blindness,* records the long onset of blindness and his gradual acceptance of and adaptation to this "numinous darkness," as he calls it. He writes that, except in dreams, he lost visual images—the faces of his wife and children, his own face—soon after he became completely blind at forty-eight. At first, this was an unnerving and terrible experience for him:

I find that I am trying to recall old photographs of myself, just to remember what I look like. I discover with a shock that I cannot remember. Must I become a blank on the wall of my own gallery?

To what extent is loss of the image of the face connected with loss of the image of the self? Is this one of the reasons why I often feel I am a mere spirit, a ghost, a memory?

Other people have become disembodied voices, speaking out of nowhere, going into nowhere. Am I not like this too, now that I have lost my body?

But within a couple of years, Hull arrived at a kind of peace with this loss of visual images, both old and new, becoming what he calls "a whole-body-seer." Here is his remarkable description of this new state of being: "Increasingly, I do not think of myself so much as a blind person, which would define me with reference to sighted people and as lacking something, but simply as a whole-body-seer. A blind person is simply someone in whom the specialist function of sight is now devolved upon the whole body, and no longer specialized in a particular organ. Being a WBS is to be in one of the concentrated human conditions."

Oliver Sacks gives a neurological explanation for Hull's experience. Neuroscientists have discovered that the visual cortex, the part of the brain that usually processes visual stimuli, doesn't shrivel up or die in blind people, but instead is "reallocated" to interpret sound, smell, taste, touch, thoughts, emotions. Sacks writes: "What happens when the visual cortex is no longer limited, or constrained, by any visual input? The simple answer is that, isolated from the outside, the visual cortex becomes hypersensitive to internal stimuli of all sorts: its own autonomous activity; signals from other brain areas—auditory, tactile, and verbal areas; and the thoughts and emotions of the blinded individual." Sacks says that Hull has "extricate[d] himself from visual nostalgia, from the strain, or falsity, of trying to pass as 'normal.' " Hull and many others challenge the idea that when we lose the ability to see and to imagine visually, we also lose our ability to think, learn, and live in an ever-expanding world.

But many people who go blind, especially those who think in intensely visual images, choose the opposite path, in a sense feeding and sharpening their visual imaginations rather than shifting to a world made primarily of sounds and textures. One of these people is an Australian psychologist named Zoltan Torey, a refugee from Soviet Hungary who was instantaneously blinded in a chemical accident. In his memoir, *Out of Darkness,* he describes his horror of "the empty darkness" that had descended upon him and his determination to use all the resources of memory and imagination in addition to new learning to build an inner world rich with color, shapes, proportion, and light. He tested his inner world for accuracy against the outside world, sometimes in harrowing ways, at least for his neighbors who saw a blind man up on his roof, making repairs in the dark. He used his formidable powers of visualization to see the meshing of gears in gear boxes, the inner workings of cells, and the brain, which he imagines as "a perpetual juggling act of interacting routines."

Blind artists may also choose to cultivate their visual imaginations. One of them is painter Lisa Fittipaldi. She had been a nurse and then a CPA when she became blind at forty-eight. She had never drawn or painted, but painting became her way out of despair and rage. She developed a system of staples and grids to situate herself on the canvas and excavated memory and fresh experiences to create oil paintings that are realistic in form but surrealistic in their light- and color-drenched brilliance. She says that learning to be at home in the world of the canvas helped her feel at home again in the big world she thought she had lost forever. Another artist is my nephew Chad, who, from the time he could hold a pencil and draw lines and shapes, wanted to be an architect. Instead of following the counsel of those who urged him to choose a less visually demanding field, Chad stuck to what he believes is his vocation, using his innate sense of space and his perfect pitch to design buildings that are both visually and acoustically pleasing.

Both he and Jeb say that their minds and imaginations fill in what they can't see.

As Oliver Sacks is quick to point out, and as our experience tells us, no person's imagination is tethered to just one sense, insofar as we understand how the imagination works. I've been asking these questions about imagination not to arrive at a definitive answer or to urge blind people in one direction or another but to move toward another question: What does blindness do to a person's ability to make the imaginative leap we call "compassion" or "empathy," the ability to leave the confined country of our own lives and step into strange worlds? Does physical blindness close the mind and heart to the happiness and pain of others, or does it open them wide? Two of the figurative definitions of 'blind,' "inconsiderate" and "lacking affect," raise and seem to answer these questions.

Two of my sisters felt invisible to my dad. Elaine says that every day in grade school she sat quietly at her desk and prayed for the miracle of sight. She hoped against hope and reason that one day she'd go home and Dad would be able to see. Mona, the youngest, born when Dad's eyesight was all but gone, also felt invisible. He couldn't see her, and, worse yet, he couldn't seem to imagine who she was. But to Darrel Kline, a blind friend of my parents who became Mona's lifelong friend and protector, she was a rainbow; and Darrel was a rainbow to her, a funny, practical, talkative, opinionated, loving man, who also happened to be blind. Darrel had no children of his own, and he became for Mona the dad our father couldn't be for her.

In reflecting on their blindness, some say that the thing they miss most is faces and smiles. Eric Weihenmayer says, "I miss looking into people's eyes, and I miss seeing their expressions change from sad to happy, from anger to laughter." John Hull writes about his four-year-old daughter trying to put into words what he calls "the breakdown which blindness causes in the language of smiles," as she wonders how he knows when to smile at her since he can't see her smiling at him. Hull says that after he became blind, a smile became a decision rather than a natural response: "You smile spontaneously when you receive a smile. For me, it is like sending off dead letters." Though one of my warmest memories of my dad is of his great, whole-hearted laugh, he, too, gradually forgot to smile.

Still, I trace to him as well as to our mother a love for anyone small, suffering, or beaten down. I suspect that my brother and sisters would say the same. Our mother was a loving woman whose generosity reached far beyond her family, though she was so quiet about it that we discovered it almost by chance. For years she volunteered at the St. Vincent de Paul Society in Mandan, sorting, mending, and pricing donated clothes to be sold to people who were down on their luck. She took old furry coats and transformed them into Winnie-the-Pooh, Tigger, and other fanciful creatures to be distributed at Christmas. She knit hundreds of pairs of mittens, and when she suffered the heart attack that killed her, she was knitting a sock of many-colored scraps of yarn, a frugal rainbow for a child with cold feet.

My dad's temper, depression, and silence sometimes blotted out his tenderness, but each of us remembers times when he sensed pain, need, or embarrassment and hurried to ease it. He cried harder than Jeanne did when she fell on St. Joseph grade school's concrete steps and broke off her two front teeth, permanent ones, leaving bloody stumps in the middle of her beautiful smile. When Jeanne had the mumps and couldn't eat, he brought her Whiz bars, sweet concoctions of chocolate over soft marshmallow that would slide down easily. Jeanne also remembers that he was kind to drunks and other undesirables. She told me a story I had forgotten: "One night we were eating supper and a very drunk man came to the door, wanting to call for a ride. Dad not only let him in the house, but helped him so he wouldn't fall on the steps. I always thought he would have helped anyone." He sold groceries on credit to men who never had and never would pay their bills, because they had hungry kids at home.

When I imagine the eventual loss of my eyesight, I dread the day when I can no longer pick up the trails of feeling, thought, and sensation that crisscross a room. I dread being on the sidelines of the wordless dance that goes on wherever people gather: the laughter at a funny move or look, the quiet smile moving around the room like the light from a candle flame, the play of emotion on faces, conspiratorial glances, silent tears. Will my face, too, forget how to open in listening, soften in response, relax when tension melts into laughter? How will I know what people are feeling, when I can't catch their slightest falling into grief? For someone who lives in her eyes as I do and as my dad did, this is a death.

But it's not the death of the mind and heart that the language of blindness imagines. In fact, the growing number of men and women who speak and write honestly and brilliantly about their experiences of blindness have convinced me that the opposite is true: that blind people can teach everyone a new kind of vision and a new kind of compassion and that together we can imagine and create a planet of the blind where everyone will be welcome.

In fact, the Planet of the Blind already exists, at least out in the cosmos of Stephen Kuusisto's imagination. Here is this wonderful place, a witty counterweight to the Kingdom of the Blind Saramago invented:

> On the planet of the blind, no one needs to be cured. Blindness is another form of music, like the solo clarinet in the mind of Bartók.

On the planet of the blind, the citizens live in the susurrus
of cricket wings twinkling in inner space.

You can hear the stars on the windless nights of June.

On the planet of the blind, people talk about what they do
not see, like Wallace Stevens, who freely chased tigers in
red weather. Here, mistaken identities are not the stuff of
farce. Instead, unvexed, the mistaken discover new and
friendly adjacent arms to touch.

On this particular planet, the greyhounds get to snooze at
last in the tall grass.

The sighted are beloved visitors, their fears of blindness
assuaged with fragrant reeds. On the planet of the blind,
everyone is free to touch faces, paintings, gardens—even
the priests who have come here to retire.

There is no hunger in the belly or in the eyes.

And the furniture is always soft. Chairs and tables are never
in the way.

On the planet of the blind, the winds of will are fresh as a
Norwegian summer. And the sky is always between moon-
shine and morning star.

God is edible.

On the planet of the blind self-contempt is a museum.

Crossing the vast space separating this imagined planet from the
hard-edged, fast-paced, sight-obsessed world we live in calls for the
greatest empathetic imagination on the part of people who can see,
those who can't, and everyone in between.

In fact, several revolutionary changes are already in the making,
although they're still largely hidden from sight. One of these has
to do with our understanding of vision. Neuroscientists now know
that vision requires more than healthy eyes and light. It happens

in the brain, which, from birth, has to learn to make sense of the oddly shaped splotches of color hitting the retina, has to learn distance and perspective, the movement of objects in space, and the body's relationship to those objects. People blind from birth or from a very early age who regain their sight through surgery struggle mightily to learn to see the world; some give up the struggle, preferring the grace, comfort, and self-confidence of the world they knew through their other senses. People who go blind later in life lose their eyesight but not necessarily their vision. An article describing an exhibit by blind artists at Berkeley says that at this moment "traditional meanings of vision and blindness are giving way": "It seems [that] a healthy brain is capable of representing line, color and perspective from a variety of sources, not merely from eyesight. This means that a sightless person can see and that a sightless person with artistic ability can give a powerful, organized representation of reality in a way that an artist with intact eyesight normally wouldn't. And because the optic eye fixes on objects and on the boundaries between things, some say the inner eye sees wider." We know for sure that even people with perfect vision are impaired and even blind if we consider the full spectrum of available light. As astronomy professor Bernard Beck-Winchatz says, "We're all blind to x-rays. We're all blind to radio waves." There's no reason, he says, why a blind person can't be a research astronomer, since we're all blind to the far reaches of the universe. Beck-Winchatz explains that "over the last 50 to 100 years . . . most astronomy research has shifted from the frequency of 'visible light' of objects that can be seen to frequencies that can only be detected by scientific instruments." My nephew Jeb reminds us that everyone sees the same narrow band of light that he sees, even though he's legally blind. He says: "Interestingly, if we could see the entire spectrum, some people might say that their favorite color is Radar or maybe X-ray, instead of, say, blue. Those other colors are out there, but we just don't receive that information. This is a visual impairment that all of us have."

Another revolutionary change is in the attitudes toward abilities and disabilities of all kinds, reflected in laws, discoveries, inventions, and technological developments. Like all people with disabilities, blind people ask that the sighted world abandon pity and paternalism and consider them equal partners with equal rights and responsibilities who know what they need and can help create it. The simple but powerful first principle of the international disability movement—"Nothing about us without us"—has helped make the world of the blind and visually impaired safer, more expansive, more secure, and more exciting. Here are a few examples. When my nephews were in their twenties, night vision scopes developed by the army let them see the starry sky for the first time. Bech-Winchatz has collaborated with astronomer Norene Grice to produce *Touch the Universe: A NASA Braille Book of Astronomy*, which puts under the fingertips of blind readers fourteen Hubble photographs of galaxies and nebulae. It's now possible to equip homes with appliances controlled by a voice-activated computer; and self-guided cars—true automobiles—are on the drawing board, though most people would prefer accessible, prompt, regular, affordable public transportation. A relatively new but promising idea is the development of universal architectural, environmental, and product designs that make homes and public spaces equally accessible to everyone, without calling attention to disabilities. A simple example are the motion-sensor lights Jeb's father installed in the hallways of their home. These friendly lights certainly make it easier for Jeb to navigate, but everyone welcomes them and is glad not to have to fumble for light switches in the dark.

Some new ideas are both simple and brilliant and take into account not just physical needs but emotional and intellectual ones as well. For eighty years wonderful people who understand both animals and blindness have trained guide dogs, matching up a dog with a human companion and then training the pair of them. But dogs, especially big ones, have a short life span, and many blind people know that they'll have to face the death of a beloved guide and companion, maybe several times during their life. A few years ago Janet and Don Burleson began training miniature horses as guides. Barring accidents, the little horses live thirty to forty years rather than ten or twelve and are as reliable and steady as dogs, with unerring memories for place and direction. Besides, they're cheap to maintain, munching on grass and a few bucketsful of oats a year. Dan Shaw was the first person to be paired up with a guide horse, a pretty little mare named Cuddles, who wears sneakers for traction and attracts a lot of attention when she and Dan take a plane or the New York subway. Dan wrote about her in a *Newsweek* article, saying that she has given him back the freedom, self-confidence, and contact with the world that his progressive eye disease had taken away.

Private, local, national, and international organizations ensure that blind and visually impaired people know what resources exist, teach them to use those resources, and develop new technologies and teaching strategies. The biggest and most well known in the United States are the National Federation of the Blind, the American Foundation for the Blind, and the Foundation Fighting Blindness. Other small ones are also doing important work. For instance, the Mind's Eye Foundation, founded by painter Lisa Fittipaldi, provides state-of-the-art technology to deaf, blind, and visually impaired children. Because the foundation is small, privately funded, and flexible, it matches up kids and machines quickly, with a minimum of red tape; the machines go with the children from home to school and back.

But technology is only a partial answer for people with disabilities, no matter what the disability is; and in many parts of the world, it's no answer at all. Imagination, once again, has to take us past the boundaries of our technologically sophisticated world, where people with money and instant access to information and training can take advantage of these astounding inventions and programs. But the World Health Organization estimates that 90 percent of the world's 37 million blind people live in the poorest parts of the developing world. For them, talking computers, hand-held readers, and closed-circuit television would be worse than useless, even if the people could afford them. In his wonderful book, *A Matter of Dignity: Changing the World of the Disabled,* Andrew Potok describes the work of people such as John Fago, who teaches people in Mexico, Cambodia, and Uganda to make artificial legs and arms out of padded leather cuffs, scrap wood, car tires, PVC pipe, and bamboo, some of these parts rescued from construction sites and garbage dumps. Alex Truesdell makes chairs for disabled children "out of cardboard, papier-mâché, and glue," in New York, India, and parts of South America. Potok, who is blind and also an artist and writer, comments that low-tech, human solutions are always crucial, "certainly not excluding the articulate human voice describing the visual world. Going to a museum can still be an immense pleasure if the person I'm with is an imaginative, informed talker."

Maybe even more important are the simple, everyday acts of imagination expressed in the Blind Beatitudes. Here are few of them:

Blessed are they who talk directly to me and not to someone else.

Blessed are they who say who they are when they enter a room and say goodbye to me when they leave so I am not left speaking to the air.

Blessed are they who wait for me to extend my hand in greeting.

Blessed are they who place my hand on an object such as
the back of a chair when telling me where it is, so that I
can seat myself.

Blessed are they who come up to me in a large crowd and
offer to help when I appear disorientated.

Blessed are they who do not leave me in a strange environ-
ment without orienting me to it.

Blessed are they who offer me an arm so they can serve as
my guide, instead of grabbing, pulling, or shoving me.

Blessed are they who read me the menu and its prices and let
me order my own meal, and then take me to the cashier
so I can pay for it.

Blessed are they who do not distract my guide dog from
being my active eyes.

Blessed are they who treat me like a human being.

These Beatitudes call for common sense and common courtesy
rather than unusual delicacy.

I see one more way in which blindness may stifle imagination
rather than increasing its reach and daring. I wonder whether the
physical hazards created by poor vision make you long for all kinds
of safety, even in your mind, where you're afraid to step too close
to the edge. The external world is a dark unknown, mined with
hazards—sidewalks that fold and ripple; walls, doors, sharp corners
that leap out suddenly where there should be open air; cars that
come screaming around corners or run red lights just when you
thought it was safe to cross the street; dogs, cats, and children who
materialize underfoot, even though you drag your feet rather than
striding boldly through space. Do you then learn to stay in the
rooms of the past, ones with no dark corners and no surprises or
challenges you'll be tempted to take on? My sister Coreen didn't
see well enough to drive when her children were young. She was

a single mother, living in Missoula, Montana, where mountain ranges rise tantalizingly on every horizon. Yellowstone and Glacier Parks are only a few hours away. She longed to go camping with her kids, but there was no public transportation to any of the parks or mountain ranges; on Sunday, even the city buses stopped running, so they could go only where their feet or bikes could take them. She wanted to go on adventures with her children, but many of those adventures weren't possible. Did she become reluctant to dream, knowing that she couldn't make even modest dreams come true?

I'm convinced that Jacques Lusseyran, a hero of the French resistance, was right when he said that it wasn't blindness but anger, bitterness, and fear that sometimes darkened his inner vision and snuffed out his compassion. When he was free from those emotions, he was also free to distinguish loyal members of the resistance from traitors and to lay a comforting hand on the people dying all around him at Buchenwald. I know that my dad was often bitter, angry, and afraid; maybe that's why he couldn't always see his children and let them know he loved them or let his world expand beyond the safety of our home. Almost every blind person whose story I've read admits to feeling despair, apathy, envy, self-pity, and fury at God, parents, and people who can see. All of them admit to fear. These feelings rise in waves that threaten to drown them in sorrow and loss. Stephen Kuusisto writes of one low period in his life, "I envy all who see things. The goddamned bird-watchers, motorcycle riders, butterfly collectors, I envy them all. . . . I envy and envy and envy." My sister Coreen usually refuses to let her fading eyesight determine her happiness, saying, "No matter how frustrated I get, there is no one I would rather be, no life I would rather have." Still, some experiences plunge her into fury: "I remember walking home from school in the dark one

winter night. I misjudged a step; my legs went out behind me.
I can still feel my chin bouncing on the sidewalk. I cried all the
way home. When I got in the house I yelled and screamed, hating
myself and my whole lot in life."

But blind people aren't the only ones who let fear keep them
from imagining new worlds. I often hear people say, "I just can't
imagine what it would be like to be homeless; a victim of rape
or incest; an Iraqi or Lebanese or Somali mother grieving for
her children; crippled, deaf, blind." When I and others say these
words, I suspect that what we really mean is that we don't want
to imagine these extreme though very common situations because
they present such harrowing challenges to our consciences and to
our notions of what it means to be human. The wonderful thing
I've discovered is that some people are striding past their fears and
imagining their way into sorrows and disabilities of all kinds. Some
take the even braver step of facing down our culture's old, false
notions of normalcy and physical and mental perfection, recogniz-
ing that there is an infinite number of ways to be human. This is
what every disability, every difference, every divergence from the
norm demonstrates. In *Blindness,* the doctor's sharp-eyed wife says,
"Perhaps humanity will manage to live without eyes, but then it will
cease to be humanity." The imaginative, brave people I'm talking
about, whether sighted or blind, know or at least suspect that the
opposite is true: that being blind is a chance to learn something
about being human we can't know in any other way. Certainly, we
must learn how to be blind and pass our knowledge on. But we
must also learn the wisdom blindness holds at its core, a wisdom
we can't arrive at by any other route.

NINE

Blind

To dazzle, to dim by excess of light, to eclipse

Y DAD, DENNIS FAULKNER, died on February 8, 1966, and was buried on a bitter winter day. After the small crowd of friends and relatives had gone home, the young parish priest brought his guitar to our house, and we sang for hours, ending with "Galway Bay," one of Dad's favorite songs. Then we scattered, each of us dealing with our memories in silence and solitude. Though we've always been a storytelling family, in the forty years since his death, we haven't told each other the stories that would keep him alive in our common memory. Nor have we created a mythology about him to pass on to the next generations as so many families do. Some of the stories in this book come from my memory and a few more from those precious old letters. But I heard many of them for the first time in recent conversations with my sisters and brother, conversations we wouldn't have had except for this book's insistent questions. I see traces of my dad in all of us, in the way we sit and stand and walk, in our quick anger and gut-splitting laughter, in the music we carry in our heads and feet, in our pride in being Irish, our skepticism, our sensitivity to injustice. My dad's blindness, too, has lived on in five of us, though the wisdom it may have taught him seems to have followed him to the grave.

I've been writing this book, or preparing to write it, all my life, long before I knew that I, too, have retinitis pigmentosa and might one day be blind. Ten years ago, when I finally put the first words on paper, I had a constricted and tragic view of blindness. When I look back on my early notes for the book, I'm shocked at their narrowness and inaccuracy. For there, in all their shameful glory, are most of the patronizing and damaging misconceptions, stereotypes, and bad attitudes I've tried to dismantle in these chapters. How could I have lived with visual impairments and blindness all my life and learned so little about and from them? The answer, I think, lies in the silence—our dad's, ours. Silence, like darkness, is a wonderful thing, but if you can't say out loud what you think and feel, you can't find out how right- or wrong-headed you are. Research for this book has been a short course in the humility necessary to correct the narrowness of individual memory and perception. I was wrong about blindness and blind people, as well as about the host of other people and events blindness led me to: the Famine Irish, the Mandan Indians and the Garrison Dam, the Germans from Russia. I may still be partially wrong about some of these happenings, but now I can find that out, as my family and others read what I have to say.

In the beginning I said to myself that I was setting out to find the gifts in blindness, something my dad wouldn't or couldn't do. Back then, I meant physical blindness. But the search for gifts has widened like a river in flood time, and it now carries in its slow-moving, life-giving waters all the kinds of blindness the language has washed up. I'll make my way to those other kinds of blindness by way of literal blindness, whose generosity is as contradictory and changeable as everything else about it. A few blind people would proclaim with Jacques Lusseyran, "For more than thirty-five years now I have been blind, completely blind. I know that this experience is my greatest happiness. . . . I know, too, that it is not my privilege, my property, but a gift that I must accept anew every day, and that all the blind can receive in their own way." Most blind people make more tentative and often contradictory claims. Blind artist Lisa Fittipaldi, for instance, says that blindness taught her what she hadn't been able to learn as a hard-driving, successful sighted person: "I truly feel that unless blindness had toppled the carefully maintained edifice I called my life, there's no way that I would be the kinder, more fulfilled person I am today. I found my life's passion in painting. Blindness took away my sight but gave me the clarity of vision. It took blindness to teach me the meaning of love and friendship." But she also calls blindness "an imposition." John Howard Griffin often thanked God for the gifts of blindness and eventual paralysis; but a few months after his sight unexpectedly returned, he opened a storeroom and came upon the dark glasses he used to wear. He was shocked by the sight and even more by his reaction: "All the horror of those past years exploded, smothering me. . . . I wanted desperately to take those glasses and throw them away with that film of dust on them . . . I saw the cane, too, but that did not matter. Only those terrible black glasses casting a dust-blurred highlight burned in my consciousness. They looked blind, staring."

For John Hull blindness is the "wrapping" of a gift that lies on the other side, one he didn't ask for and would never wish on his children. On the Planet of the Blind Stephen Kuusisto has found beauty and deep empathy, "roses grow[ing] on the sheer banks of the sea cliff." But he also wanted so badly to see "the damned birds" that he went into a deserted university ornithology lab and found an open specimen case. He took out the birds one by one and held them close to his face, wondering all the while what he'd say if a security guard should come by. Perhaps, "I'm blind, sir, and this is my first experience with birds!" Finally, in a hilarious account of his struggles with RP, a young Canadian teacher named Ryan Knighton says, "People often ask me what I hate most about blindness. *Blindness* is the answer—I hate blindness most about blindness." To satisfy the people who don't like that answer, he adds, "The public john proves, once and for all, that hell for the blind is made of porcelain." Still, he laughs at his misadventures and entices his readers to laugh with him.

The fact that more and more visually impaired and blind people write about their experience has convinced me that there are many gifts in acknowledging blindness. The first practical gifts are the many adaptations others have developed and willingly pass on. The second is the blessed knowledge that you're not alone, even in your denial, your efforts to pass for a sighted person, your subterfuges. Out in the open, there can be a community of the blind and places where they meet to talk and laugh with understanding but without pity. People who are openly blind become teachers. When Stephen Kuusisto ventures out with his guide dog, strangers want to talk to him about their newly blind wife or friend or student. In addition, people who are frankly and openly blind can help those who depend on vision realize what they're missing, as well as what they have. For instance, in 2005, a restaurant owner in Paris opened a restaurant called "Dans le Noir," "In Blackness." Blind waiters guide sighted diners into cavelike darkness where they experience both the limited and the heightened sensitivity blindness confers. As a reporter says, "Fingertips seek out familiarity, patting the table for a fork, a plate, a hand to hold. The nose perks up to every passing plate. Under cover of darkness, texture and shape take on new importance. One realizes the role sight plays in the joy of eating."

While some diners are not thrilled by the experience and declare the food mediocre and the whole idea a marketing scam, I see Dans le Noir as a sensual expression of an intellectual, emotional, and spiritual reality. In spite of our best efforts to act rationally, with what we call "insight" and "foresight," in many of life's most important and dangerous moments, we must go blind or not go at all. Loving anyone or anything; bearing and raising children; believing in people, institutions, God; teaching; research in any field that goes beyond the edge of the known world and its maps; grief, confusion, loss, death—all dark caves where the sighted have no advantages over the blind.

The dictionary as well as events of the second half of the twentieth century remind us that light isn't always the good that the book of Genesis celebrates. It can be blinding and painful, as well as illuminating, as in *blinding flash* and *snow-blind.* Several languages have had to coin new words to say that light can also be deadly in ways people of earlier centuries couldn't have imagined. *The American Heritage Dictionary of the English Language* informs us that *Blitzkrieg,* "lightning-war," comes from the same Indo-European root as *blind.* The survivors of the atomic bombs the United States dropped on Hiroshima and Nagasaki in 1945, bombs with the brightness of ten thousand suns, call themselves *hibakusha,* which one might translate "survivors of the light." And who can forget the seductively beautiful tracer rounds of artillery and the smart bombs exploding brilliantly over Afghanistan and Iraq in our recent televised wars, or the television itself, an eye always wide open and watching?

The excess of light, or maybe the follies committed in the light, make some people yearn for darkness and the blessings of sightlessness. One of these is Black Elk, the Oglala Sioux holy man John D. Neihardt interviewed in the early 1930s and whose life and vision for the Indian people Neihardt recorded in *Black Elk Speaks*. Black Elk was almost blind when Neihardt met him at Pine Ridge Reservation in South Dakota. His Messianic dream for his people had faded, as the United States government made and broke treaties; white settlers, hunters, and prospectors destroyed the buffalo herds and laid claim to the gold in the Black Hills; and his people, penned up on reservations, starved. Worst of all, Black Elk had seen "a people's dream that died in bloody snow" in the 1890 massacre at Wounded Knee, when the U.S. cavalry pursued fleeing women and children and killed them. It's no wonder that Black Elk preferred blindness to "the darkness of men's eyes."

Black Elk, like many other poets and prophets, knew that wonderful things happen in the dark and can't happen without it. Seeds stir and fatten in dark soil. In the seething, decaying centers of compost heaps, new soil forms; and narcissus and night-blooming cereus blossom only at night. In wombs, human babies, like nocturnal animals, live in darkness, navigating by taste, touch, hearing, and smell. Sometimes people with sight deliberately choose darkness or limited vision. We dim the house lights at a concert so that we can hear the music more purely. Skilled diagnosticians sometimes close their eyes as their hands explore the terrain of bodies. We listen for frightening, exotic, and beautiful night sounds: the wide-winged moth at the screen, the secret language of loons, the sudden loud rustle in the grass. Every spring people from all over the world flock to the sand flats of the Platte River near Kearney, Nebraska, for a sensory experience remarkably similar to retinitis pigmentosa. They come to see the migration of a half million sandhill cranes, gray birds with golden beaks and a wing span of six or seven feet. From dusk to deepest dark, the watchers huddle in wooden blinds with peepholes. They wait in absolute silence, able to see only what's directly in front of them—the endless procession of the great birds as they prepare for sleep—and to hear in the silence the breathing of the people around them, the birds calling to family members, and the occasional thunder of wings when an eagle comes in and spooks them. The most restorative sleep, the sleep that yields dreams, happens in deepest darkness. In fact, darkness is good for all kinds of dreaming. When I was about seven years old, I used to escape every summer day after noon dinner to our playhouse, an old chicken coop that still held the smells of eggs and hatching chicks. I sat on a splintery two-by-eight plank with a warped curve in the middle. With the door shut and only a few rifts of dusty light, it was too dark to read or play, but that wasn't what I'd come to do. To myself I called this my dreaming time. I needed to shut out the bright, dry sun, so high in the sky it didn't cast a shadow, so that I could follow my imagination wherever it lead. Even as a child I knew that beauty and mystery grow in the darkness.

You'd think, then, that for me physical blindness would be a gift because it takes away the temptation to escape into light. But darkness and blindness aren't the same, though our language often tricks us into thinking they are. It seems to me that most of us who love the dark love it, in part, because we know it's not eternal. The earth turns, the seasons shift, and even the longest night yields to day. The days lengthen after seemingly endless northern winters, and suddenly it's spring: seeds are growing toward the sun, and babies are traveling blind and bundled from the darkness of the womb through the birth canal to discover sight and all its blooming wonders. Every day I emerged from the chicken coop, my dreaming place, into the light where I could read, watch spider webs flicker in the sun, and be another pair of eyes for my dad. Jacques Lusseyran writes about "the despotism of sight," arguing that flickering, flighty visual stimuli keep us from a deeper knowledge of reality that our other senses and our imaginations can lead us to. But some of us love and will always long for the hard-edged world of sight, filled, yes, with pain and ugliness, but also with a frayed, imperfect beauty.

Love of light and all it reveals and blesses makes me hope and pray for cures. I want doctors around the world to prevent the 75 percent of blindness that is already preventable. I also want a cure for retinitis pigmentosa or at least a treatment that will slow down its shadowy progress. I watch for news of bionic eyes, drug delivery systems, retinal transplants, and genetic engineering that will help not only people with RP but also the millions with macular degeneration, diabetic retinopathy, and the amazing range of other eye diseases. But I know from all these decades of waiting that a treatment or cure might not happen in my lifetime or even the lifetimes of my nephews and grandnephews. I have concluded that we daren't enslave ourselves to hope. To borrow one more time from Tillie Olsen, we have to live as fully as possible and keep challenging any structures or attitudes that "will not let life be" for blind or visually impaired people, ourselves and the people who would not be cured even by the breakthroughs barely visible on the far horizon.

Is it possible to hope for sight, pray for it, work for it and still believe and insist that being "normal" isn't all it's cracked up to be? That's a precarious balancing act, but there are grave dangers in not putting ourselves in that position. My reflections on blindness have forced me to rethink many things, including my images of God and of the kingdom of God. When my dad died, I imagined him waking up with a whole eternity ahead of him to see what he'd been missing on earth. My image of heaven was like that of a South African man I recently heard of who grew up under apartheid. His elders taught him that if he was a good, obedient boy, when he died he'd go to heaven and be white, because the blood of the Lamb would wash away not his sins but his blackness. But as many people with disabilities now say, maybe God, too, is disabled, or at least a God of the disabled, as much darkness as light; and maybe in the family of God the only norms are justice and mercy. To be a member of this ragtag family, you don't need to be white, male, heterosexual, beautiful, athletic, thin, tan, middle-class. You don't need to be able to see.

I've been thinking and writing about many kinds of blindness and now wonder whether they, too, are gifts rather than the disastrous human tendencies I've always pictured. Can it be that blind prejudice, the blind eye we turn on injustice, the blindness of ideology, the sighted world's inability to see the blind all have crucial lessons to teach? I recently heard Basil Braveheart, a Lakota teacher and healer who lives on the Pine Ridge Reservation in South Dakota, talk about his efforts to conquer the alcoholism that began after he returned from the Korean War. He and his fellow soldiers had committed terrible atrocities against Chinese prisoners, and he drank to dim the nightmares. He tried many conventional recovery methods, but all of them, he says, tried to wipe out the disease or at least "put it in a closet" where it would be out of sight. He became sober when he turned to an old spiritual teaching of the Lakota. Whenever you are dealing with a powerful, destructive energy, that spirituality teaches, you need to honor it and acknowledge it as a cousin and a friend. Every morning Basil Braveheart sits down with his alcoholism and listens. He says that alcoholism "has been my most prolific teacher. It tells me each morning who I am. I honor it."

Maybe the gift I've been looking for in physical blindness and its many figurative relatives is the courage to face every day what I and past generations have hidden away and silenced. I wondered ten years ago whether my father, Dennis Faulkner, would lead me after him, cursing, into the darkness. I worried that my questions would chafe old hurts in me and in my sisters and brother that no words could soothe. As I sat down with my memories of him day after day, he did lead me into the darkness, not with a curse but with a blessing.

Recently, three generations of our family came from all parts of the country to gather in Mandan, not at our home place but in the hills west of town where Elaine lives in an earth-sheltered home she and her husband designed and built. It's surrounded by flower beds and gardens like our mom's that lure butterflies and birds. One night we sat outside in the long North Dakota twilight, telling stories, playing the fiddle and the harmonica, dancing a wild jig, and singing old songs. One of our favorites, naturally, was an Irish song, and we repeated its brave, hopeful refrain: "The cares of tomorrow must wait till this day is done." The cares rose up in and around us: the tumor growing in my brother Dennie's brain, the diminishing eyesight we'd told each other about earlier that day, the worries, troubles, and sorrows that afflict every family, the stubborn blindness perpetuating war and terror in our world. Still, we sang, as our dad had taught us to, until full darkness fell and the new moon rose over the hills.

When we were young, Dad used to come into the house at night after a long day at work in the market, carrying a bucket of ice cold well water. Then, like a magician, he produced from his overall pockets apples he had shined up just for us, his kids. If it had been a good day, and he was feeling frisky, he sang a bit of song and did a quick step dance on the kitchen linoleum. I think often of his advice, "Learn all you can, kids," and the questions he asked to the day he died. Water, apples, music, questions—those caves in our knowledge that pull us into deepest darkness. Gifts to hold and then pass on.

Notes

Chapter 1

3   "imprisoned . . .": Germaine Greer, interview with Joseph Kastner, ed. Janet Todd, *Women Writers Talking* (New York: Holmes and Meier, 1983), 144.

10   It was a dazzling surprise: *American Heritage Dictionary of the English Language*, 4th ed. (New York: Houghton Mifflin, 2000), 2022–23.

11   In the constellation: Robert L. Chapman, ed., *Roget's International Thesaurus*, 5th ed. (New York: HarperCollins, 1992).

12   "It is imperative . . .": Antonio Gramsci, qtd in Edward W. Said, *Orientalism* (New York: Pantheon, 1978), 25 and note pp. 329–30.

12   "a good memoir is also . . .": William Zinsser, ed., Introduction, *Inventing the Truth: The Art and Craft of Memoir* (Boston: Houghton Mifflin, 1998), 15.

13   "communal memoir": Patricia Hampl, "Memory and Imagination," in *I Could Tell You Stories* (New York: Norton, 1999), 36.

Chapter 2

18   "My father's harmonica . . .": Jeanne Adelmeyer, unpublished poem.

20   "the hidden injuries . . .": Tillie Olsen, *Silences* (New York: Feminist Press, 2003), 263.

24   breadwinners for the family: Janet A. Nolan, *Ourselves Alone: Women's Emigration from Ireland 1885–1920* (Lexington, Kentucky: University Press of Kentucky, 1989), 81.

24   "a professional nurse": *Alexandria Citizen,* 18 May 1905.

28   "A disabled adult man . . .": John M. Hull, *Touching the Rock: An Experience of Blindness* (New York: Pantheon Books, 1990), 106.

28   "marginalized as a father . . .": Hull, 62.

28   closed to him: Hull, 186–87.

28   "I still have difficulty . . .": Hull, 115–16.

29   "That is what I like . . .": Erik Weihenmayer, *Touch the Top of the World: A Blind Man's Journey to Climb Farther Than the Eye Can See* (New York: Dutton, 2001), 283.

30   "testosterone levels . . .": Weihenmayer, 87–88.

30   "Some people think . . .": Weihenmayer, 144–45.

31   revealed her weight to him: Weihenmayer, 286–87.

31   "It worried me . . .": Robert V. Hine, *Second Sight* (Berkeley: University of California Press, 1993), 166.

37   "share want": Olsen, "I Stand Here Ironing," in *Tell Me a Riddle* (New York: Delta/Seymour Laurence, 1989), 2.

38   "In this universe . . .": Mary Oliver, "The Bright Eyes of Eleonora: Poe's Dream of Recapturing the Impossible," in *Winter Hours:*

Prose, Prose Poems, and Poems (Boston: Houghton Mifflin, 1999), 48.

Chapter 3

40   "I found it easy . . .": Hine, 189.

40   "You think dark . . .": Toni Morrison, *Song of Solomon* (New York: Penguin Books, 1977), 40.

40   According to the World Health Organization: "Vision 2020: the Right to Sight," 7 January 2008, <http:www.v2020.org>.

43   "Blindness has not . . .": Jorge Luis Borges, "Blindness," in *The Art of the Personal Essay*, ed. Phillip Lopate (New York: Anchor Books, 1994), 381.

43   "overcome blindness": Borges, 385.

45   "accurately threaded . . .": Olsen, "Requa," *Iowa Review* 1, no. 3 (Summer 1970): 71–72.

46   "the blind have moved . . .": Kenneth Jernigan, "Blindness: Is History against Us?" 16 April 2005, <http://www.blind.net/bpbal1973.htm>.

46   "Isn't it true . . .": Jernigan.

49   "If we hear enough . . .": Kathi Wolfe, "Fighting Stereotypes: 'Supercrips' Images Pose Unrealistic Expectations on Disabled People," *Minneapolis Star Tribune* 6 July 2001, 19A.

49   Besides Rachel Scdoris: "Melrose Man Braves Elements, Tests Limits at Iditarod," *St. Cloud Times,* 6 March 2005, 1B, 8B.

50   "The blind . . .": Qtd in Jacobus tenBroek and Floyd W. Matson, *Hope Deferred: Public Welfare and the Blind* (Berkeley: University of California Press, 1959), 7.

51   French makes: Qtd in tenBroek and Matson, 5–6.

51   These well-meaning experts: Qtd in tenBroek and Matson,7.

51   happened in 1957: tenBroek and Matson, 2–4.

52   "it implies total blindness . . .": Henry Grunwald, *Twilight: Losing Sight, Gaining Insight* (New York: Knopf, 1999), 87.

53   In 1995 a crew: Andrew Potok, *A Matter of Dignity: Changing the World of the Disabled* (New York: Bantam Books, 2002), 135–55.

54   "There is a blurry line . . .": *Climbing Blind Tibet Expedition*, 2004, Climbing Blind, 11 May 2005 <http://www.climbingblind. org>; Weihenmayer, 302–03.

55   "the first picture . . .": Karl Greenfeld, "Blind to Failure," *Time* 157 (June 18, 2001): 52.

55   "I did choke down . . .": Weihenmayer, 128.

55   Deborah Wingwall, one of the: Rick DelVecchio, "Blind Photographer's Vision Extends beyond her Eyes," 18 February 2005, <http://www.nfbnet.org/pipermail/artbeyondsight museums/2005/000102.html>.

55   New M.D. Tim Cordes: Susan Barnhill, "Blind Student Earns M.D.," 14 May 2005, <http://www.station504.com/BlindMD. htm>.

56   "sit around and get a tan . . .": *In the Mind of the Beholder*, Dir. Karen Brown Davison, Prod, Department of Communication, Stanford University, Videorecording, 1997.

56   "contemporary symbol . . .": Greenfeld, 5.

57   "the sighted world's . . .": Stephen Kuusisto, *Planet of the Blind* (New York: Dial Press, 1998), 161.

57 "There must have been . . .": Sally Wagner, *How Do You Kiss a Blind Girl?* (Springfield, IL: Thomas, 1986), 35.

58 In the 2000 edition: Richard Nelson Bolles, *What Color Is Your Parachute? A Practical Manual for Job-Hunters and Career Changes* (Berkeley: Ten Speed, 1990, 2000).

59 blind people could not be certified: Frederic K. Schroeder, "Orientation and Mobility, Competence and Hypocrisy," 25 July 2006, <http://www.nfb.org/bm/bm03/bm0309/Bm030908.htm>.

60 "Of course . . .": Kuusisto, 103–04.

60 There for the first time: Kuusisto, 171.

61 "on human guides . . .": Frances A. Koestler, *The Unseen Minority: A Social History of Blindness in the United States* (New York: David McKay, 1976), 304.

61 "What's the point . . .": Greenfeld, 3.

62 For example, Ginger Lee: Eric Bradley, "Disability Is No Hindrance for Blind Teacher: Blindness Enhances Her Mission to Make Children Independent," *The Braille Monitor,* May 2003, <http://www.nfb.org/bm?bm03/bm0305/bm030505.htm>.

62 "Only's": Olsen, *Silences,* 39.

63 In fact, Stephen Kuusisto: "An Interview with Stephen Kuusisto," 30 May 2005, <http://www.randomhouse.com/boldtype/0398/kuusisto/interview.html>.

63 "At the age of thirty-nine . . .": Kuusisto, 171.

63 "state-sponsored hope": Kuusisto, 181.

63 SSDI and lost taxes: *National Federation of the Blind, 2007,* 7 March 2007, <http://www.nfb.org/nfb/Default.asp>.

64 "discover the joyous striving . . .": Kuusisto, 181.

Chapter 4

72   In the 1870 Douglas County census: "United States Federal Census, 1880, 1900, 1920,"<http://www.ancestrylibrary.com/default.aspx>.

73   In his history, Karl Klein: Karl Matthias Klein, *The History of Millerville, Douglas County, Minnesota, 1866–1930* (Millerville: Klein Company Store, 1930), 10–11.

74   "Like oil lamps . . .": Eavan Boland, "The Emigrant Irish," in *An Origin Like Water: Collected Poems 1967–1987* (New York: Norton, 1996), 194.

75   and in "Famine": "Famine," in *Universal Mother Album*, 1994, Qtd in David A. Valone and Christine Kinealy, *Ireland's Great Hunger: Silence, Memory, and Commemoration* (Lanham: University Press of America, 2002), 15.

75   Forensic anthropologists: Valone and Kinealy, 101.

75   First, famine and disease: Valone and Kinealy, 2.

76   "The worst aspects . . .": Valone and Kinealy, 27.

76   "the grave of song": Qtd in Tom Hayden, *Irish on the Inside* (London: Verso, 2001), 39.

77   "Even amnesia . . .": Peter Quinn, "In Search of the Banished Children: A Famine Journey," ed. Tom Hayden, *The Irish Hunger: Personal Reflections on the Legacy of the Famine* (Boulder, CO: Roberts Rinehart, 1997), 155.

78   "a human drama . . .": Qtd in Stephen J. Campbell, *The Great Irish Famine: Words and Images from the Famine Museum, Strokestown Park, County Roscommon* (Ireland: Famine Museum, 1994), 7.

78   Cormac Ó Gráda, a careful: Cormac Ó Gráda, *The Great Irish Famine* (Cambridge: Cambridge University Press, 1995), 2.

78   By analyzing potato production: Ó Gráda, 16.

79   far from ignoring the famine: Christine Kinealy, "Potatoes, Providence and Philanthropy: The Role of Private Charity during the Irish Famine," in *The Meaning of the Famine*, vol. 6, ed. Patrick O'Sullivan (London: Leicester University Press, 1997), 144.

79   For example, the Marquis of Sligo: *When Ireland Starved*, vol. 1: "Causes of Poverty," Dir. Joseph Dunn. Videocassette, Film for the Humanities, 1993.

80   "a direct stroke . . .": James S. Donnelly, Jr., *The Great Irish Potato Famine* (Gloucestershire: Sutton, 2001), 20.

80   "the poor people . . .": Thomas Gallagher, *Paddy's Lament: Ireland 1846–1847, Prelude to Hatred* (Orlando, FL: Harcourt Brace Jovanovich, 1982), 86.

81   No one took photographs: Sean Sexton and Christine Kenealy, *The Irish: A Photohistory* (New York: Thomas and Hudson, 2002), 31, 39–61.

81   Bridget O'Donnell: Killen, 111; Donnelly, 148.

81   "mere breathing skeletons": Melissa Fegan, *Literature and the Irish Famine 1845–1919* (Oxford: Clarendon, 2002), 93.

82   "A Thousand Farewells . . .": Peatsai O'Callanan, qtd. in *Irish in America*, vol. 1.

83   the Kilrush workhouse: Donnelly 144–52; Tim Pat Coogan, "The Lessons of the Famine For Today," in Hayden, *The Irish Hunger*, 175–76.

83   The influential *London Times*: Fegan, 41, 48.

83   "influential men . . .": John W. Blassingame, ed., *The Frederick Douglass Papers*, series 1, vol. 1 (New Haven: Yale University Press, 1979–1992), 71.

83   He wrote to William: William S. McFeely, *Frederick Douglass* (New York: Norton, 1995), 126.

84   About half were illiterate: Donald Harman Akenson, *The Irish Diaspora: A Primer* (Toronto: Meany, 1993), 40.

84   County Donegal in 1837: *When Ireland Starved*, vol. 1: "Causes of Poverty."

84   Two fifths of Irish families: Quinn, 144.

85   the worst winter: Killen, 98–99.

85   "Most pitiable was . . .": Gallagher, 37.

85   chimpanzees were white: Valone and Kinealy, 239.

86   One eyewitness reports: Ó Cathaoir, frontispiece.

86   "The Famine killed everything": Valone and Kinealy, 1.

86   While Irish cottiers: Ó Cathaoir, xvi.

86   When they tried:: Donnelly, 39; Kerby Miller and Paul Wagner, *Out of Ireland: The Story of Irish Emigration to America* (Washington, DC: Elliot and Clark, 1994), 19.

86   in 1846 the Earl of Dunraven: Killen, 180.

87   Still, in 1847: Ó Cathaoir, 96.

87   "Famine Roads . . .": Eavan Boland, "Famine Roads," in Hayden, *The Irish Hunger*), 216.

87   In Black '47: *Irish in America: the Long Journey Home*, vol. 1: "The Great Hunger," Dir. Thomas Lennon & Mark Zwonitzer, Videocassette, Lennon Documentary Group, 1999.

87   "Evictions peaked . . .": Ó'Cathaoir, 167.

87   In July of 1847: Ó'Gráda, 39.

87   "instead of diggin' praties . . .": "Muirsheen Durkin," trad. *Irish Pub Classics*, Irish Records International, vol. 2, Pembroke, MA, 2001.

NOTES TO CHAPTER 4

88   *deorai—exile*: Mick Moloney, *Far from the Shamrock Shore: The Story of Irish-American Immigration through Song* (New York: Crown, 2002), 6.

88   "What compulsion . . .": Killen, 80.

88   Tens of thousands died: Cecil Woodham-Smith, *The Great Hunger: Ireland 1845–1849* (New York: Harper and Row, 1962), 252.

88   Even the good Lord Sligo of Westport: *The Irish in America,* vol. 1.

88   "Five shillings each . . .": Killen, 133–34.

88   The notorious Strokestown Castle: *Irish in America,* vol. 1.

89   It was the culmination: For a more complete history of pre-Famine Ireland, see Ann Regan, *Irish in Minnesota* (St. Paul, MN: Historical Society Press, 2002); *When Ireland Starved,* vol. 1; Luke Gibbons, "Doing Justice to the Past," in Hayden, *The Irish Hunger,* 258–70; Thomas Gallagher, *Paddy's Lament: Ireland 1846–1847, Prelude to Hatred* (Orlando, FL: Harcourt Brace Jovanovich, 1982); T. N. Moody and F. X. Martin, eds., *The Course of Irish History* (Dublin: Mercier, 1994).

90   "crowbar brigade": Donnelly, 228.

91   Because of literacy and property requirements: Campbell, 38.

91   "The judge and jury . . .": Gallagher, 53.

91   "double consciousness": W. E. B. DuBois, *The Souls of Black Folk,* ed. David W. Blight and Robert Gooding-Williams (Boston: Bedford Books, 1997), 38.

92   In New Orleans in 1853: *The Irish in America,* vol. 2: "All Across America."

92   "Irish Violence . . .": John Leo, "Of Famine and Green Beer," *U.S. News and World Report,* 122 (24 March 1997): 16.

93   the Irish used legal means: Gallagher, 290.

93   Hundreds of thousands of Irish workers: Miller, 94.

93   The obituary of my great-grandfather: *Alexandria Citizen*, 18 May 1905.

94   "if there was no hope . . .": Tom Hayden, "The Famine of Feeling," in *The Irish Hunger*, 271–93, 284–85.

95   "a form of injustice . . .": Qtd. in Gibbons, 260.

96   20,000 of them a day: Jeff Sachs, "The End of Poverty," *Time*, 11 March 2005, 46.

96   In *The Middle of Everywhere*: Mary Pipher, *The Middle of Everywhere: The World's Refugees Come to Our Town* (New York: Harcourt, 2002), 276–85, 292–304.

Chapter 5

101   "Souperism . . .": Donnelly, 234; Kinealy, 149.

106   "Recently I was up late . . .": Kuusisto, 188.

108   "Are you confident . . .": Matthew 9:27–31.

108   "I wish I could console people . . .": Kuusisto, 188–89.

109   "Creating God . . .": Helen Betenbaugh and Marjorie Procter-Smith, "Disabling the Lie: Prayers of Truth and Transformation," in *Human Disability and the Service of God: Reassessing Religious Practice*, ed. Nancy L. Eiesland and Don E. Saliers (Nashville: Abingdon, 1998), 296.

111   "Close the door . . .": Tom Springfield, "A World of Our Own," 1965.

112   They head out into the noisy upheaval: "Braille without Borders," *Climbing Blind Tibet Expedition*, 2004, Climbing Blind, 11 May 2005, <http://www.climbingblind.org/The%20Cause/braillewithoutborders.icm>.

112 "But in the Khumbu icefall . . .": Karl Greenfeld, "Blind to Failure," Time, 18 June 2001, 52.

113 "who have never hesitated . . .": Weihenmayer, n.p.

113 "There are moments . . ."; Weihenmayer, 289.

114 "Morris, you better not . . .": Weihenmayer, 290.

116 "infallible, or nearly": Jacques Lusseyran, *And There was Light: Autobiography of Jacques Lusseyran, Blind Hero of the French Resistance*, trans. Elizabeth R. Cameron (New York: Parabola Books, 1998), 176.

116 "I was carried by a hand . . .": Lusseyran, 282.

117 "in a couple years . . .": Olsen, "I Stand Here Ironing," 11.

Chapter 6

120 "irrational suspicion . . .": *Oxford English Dictionary*, < http://www.oed.com/>.

123 "This explained his jubilation . . .": John H. Griffin, *Scattered Shadows: A Memoir of Blindness and Vision* (Maryknoll, NY: Orbis Books, 2004), 164–69.

125 their long sojourn in Russia: *The Germans from Russia: Children of the Steppe, Children of the Prairie*, Producer Bob Dambach, Prairie Public Broadcasting, 1999.

126 Because Benedictine sisters had taught, nursed, and administered: Sister M. Grace McDonald, OSB, *With Lamps Burning* (Saint Joseph, MN: Saint Benedict's Priory Press, 1957), 83–84, 127–28.

127 "a paradise on the steppe": *The Germans from Russia*; Larry Batson, *The Minneapolis Tribune*, 18 June 1981, 3B, 4B.

127 the paradise lasted: *The Germans from Russia*.

129   But historians describe them: Bob Reha, "North Dakota's First Capital Punishment Case in 100 Years Set to Begin in Fargo," 13 June 2006, <http://www.minnesota.publicradio.org/display/web/2006/06/13/nddeathpenalty>

129   "One of the most misunderstood . . .": *The Germans from Russia.*

130   "Katozchki—potato eaters": Joseph S. Height, *Paradise on the Steppe: A Cultural History of the Kutschurgan, Beresan, and Liebental Colonists, 1804–1944* (Bismarck: North Dakota Historical Society of Germans from Russia, 1972), 195.

133   "curtain of censorship": John Christgau, *"Enemies": World War II Alien Internment* (Ames: Iowa State University Press, 1985), 173.

133   The men who guarded them: Christgau, vii.

134   one of eight internment centers: Jerome D. Tweton, "The Fort Lincoln Internment Camp," *North Dakota Humanities Council*, 5 February 2005, <http://www.nd-humanities.org/html/wwiiinternment.html>.

134   "Nazis and Sun Worshipers . . ." Christgau, 173.

134   "Autumn grief . . .": Itaru Ina, "Snow Country Prison: Interned in North Dakota," *North Dakota Museum of Art*, 1998, 5 February 2005, <http://www.ndmoa.com/template.cfm?page=SnowCountry Prison>.

Chapter 7

144   "1949—Three affiliated Tribes . . .": Tom Anderson, et al, eds, *Chronicle of America* (Mount Kisco, NY: Chronicle, 1989).

144   The Pick-Sloan plan: Michael L. Lawson, *Dammed Indians: The Pick–Sloan Plan and the Missouri River Sioux, 1994–1980* (Norman: University of Oklahoma Press, 1982), xxi–xxii.

146 "the most devastating effects . . .": Lawson, 27, 29.

148 In 1781 smallpox struck: Paul VanDevelder, *Coyote Warrior: One Man, Three Tribes, and the Trial that Forged a Nation* (New York: Little, Brown, 2004), 57–59.

148 The Indians welcomed the Explorers: VanDevelder, 20.

149 "sword of civilizing devastation": George Catlin, *Letter and Notes on the Manners, Customs, and Conditions of the North American Indians, Written during Eight Years' Travel (1832–39) amongst the Wildest Tribes of Indians in North America*, vols I and II (New York: Dover, 1973), 95.

149 "A better, more honest . . .": Catlin, 182.

149 "for as long as waters flow": VanDevelder, 69.

149 As early as the seventeenth century: Lawson, 8.

150 The temperature ranged: Frank H. H. Roberts, Jr. Ed., *River Basin Survey Papers: Inter-Agency Archeological Salvage Program*, vol. 6, no. 185 (Washington, DC: U.S. Government Printing Office, 1963), 11, 63.

151 "economically dependent . . .": Lawson, 33.

151 the Dawes Act: Lawson, 33.

151 "Humanitarians had long demanded . . .": Lawson, 33.

151 "sandy alluvial loam . . .": George Metcalf, "Star Village: A Fortified Historic Arikara Site in Mercer County, North Dakota," in Roberts, *River Basin Survey Papers*, 69.

152 "I am an old woman now . . .": "Waheenee: An Indian Girl's Story Told by Herself to Gilbert L. Wilson," *North Dakota History: Journal of the Northern Plains*, vol. 38, nos. 1 and 2 (Winter/Spring 1971), rpt. in Peter Nabokov, ed., *Native American Testimony* (New York: Viking, 1991), 182.

153 "Sometimes at evening . . .": "Waheenee," 182.

154   "Much more evidence . . .": George Metcalf, "Small Sites on and about Fort Berthold Indian Reservation, Garrison Reservoir, North Dakota," in Roberts, *River Basin Survey Papers*, 54.

154   "Such information . . .": Metcalf, "Small Sites," 12.

154   "reverted to their early religion": Metcalf, "Small Sites," 13.

155   "Right-of way for the Garrison Reservoir . . .": Metcalf, "Star Village," 64–65.

155   Without consulting the three tribes: VanDevelder, 105.

155   "The Flood that Stayed Forever": VanDevelder, 26, 29.

155   "fit for rattlesnakes and horned toads": VanDevelder, 118.

155   "The land beneath our feet . . .": VanDevelder, 125.

156   Understanding neither the Indians': VanDevelder, 129–33.

156   Newspapers across the country: Lauren Donovan, "Going Full Circle: Will the Return of Ancestral Lands Right an Old Wrong?" *The Bismarck Tribune*, 22 May 2005, 1A.

156   The "Taking Act" became law in 1949: VanDevelder, 139–40.

156   "For the first time . . .": VanDevelder, 159.

157   before the "Taking Act,": VanDevelder, 111–12.

158   By 1982 unemployment: VanDevelder, 238–42.

158   "They have all come to pass . . .": Carolyn Gilman and Mary Jane Schneider, *The Way to Independence* (St. Paul: Minnesota Historical Society Press, 1987), 317.

158   Fort Berthold was quickly transformed: VanDevelder, 175–76.

158   "Our thinking failed us . . .": VanDevelder, 32–33.

158   "to liberate the Indian . . .": VanDevelder, 153–54.

158   half of the Fort Berthold tribe: VanDevelder, 178.

159   In 1992, thanks to the skilled: VanDevelder, 241.

159   The tribes are now asking: Donovan, 1A, 7A.

159   The Garrison Dan, which promised: Donovan, 1A.

159   "invite us to look . . .": Campbell, 7.

160   tribes are being offered: Chris Shields, "Utah Reservation Might Store Nuclear Waste," *St. Cloud Times*, 10 September 2005, 3A.

Chapter 8

165   "The people who walked in darkness . . .": Isaiah 9:2.

165   "I am the light . . .": John 8:12.

165   "Christ, be our light . . .": Bernadette Farrell, *Christ Be Our Light* (Portland: Oregon Catholic Press, 1994).

166   "Only with the heart . . .": Antoine de Saint-Exupéry, *The Little Prince*, trans. Katherine Woods (New York: Harcourt Brace Jovanovich, 1982), 72.

166   "in unapproachable light": 1 Tim 6:16.

167   "for blindness is also this . . .": Jose Saramago, *Blindness*, trans. Giovanni Pontiero, (New York: Harcourt Brace, 1998), 188.

167   "The charitable, picturesque world . . .": Saramago, 120.

167   "nothingness trying to organize nothingness": Saramago, 228.

169   "Yeah, well, they're afraid . . .": Kuusisto, 162.

169   "Most sources of pain . . .": Jeb Willenbring, e-mail to the author, 28 June 2005.

171   Oliver Sacks, who calls himself: Oliver Sacks, "A Neurologist's Notebook: The Mind's Eye," *The New Yorker*, 28 July 2003, 51, 58–59.

173   "There's nothing left for me . . .": Horatio Nicholls and Edgar Leslie, "Among My Souvenirs," 25 October 2005, <http://www. reelclassics.com/Movies/BestYears/bestyears-souvenirs.htm>.

174   "I find that I am trying . . .": Hull, 25.

175   "Increasingly, I do not think . . .": Hull, 217.

175   Neuroscientists have discovered: Sacks, 51.

175   "What happens when . . .": Sacks, 57.

175   "extricate[d] himself . . .": Sacks, 49.

176   "perpetual juggling act . . .": Sacks, 53.

176   She had been a nurse: Lisa Fittipaldi, *A Brush with Darkness: Learning to Paint after Losing My Sight*, 14 April 2005, <http://www.andrewsmcmeel.com/products?isbn=07040746936>.

177   "I miss looking . . .": Weihenmayer, 97.

178   "You smile spontaneously . . .": Hull, 202–03, 34.

178   "One night we were eating . . .": Jeanne Adelmeyer, e-mail to the author, 28 May 2005.

179   "On the planet of the blind . . .": Kuusisto, 148.

181   "It seems [that] a healthy brain . . .": Rick DelVecchio, "Blind Photographer's Vision Extends beyond Her Eyes," 18 February 2005, <http://www.nfbnet.org/pipermail/artbeyondsight museums/2005/000102.html>.

181   "We're all blind to x-rays . . .": "Touch the Universe: Creating Cosmic Images for the Blind to 'See'," *St. Cloud Visitor* 11 September 2003.

181   "Interestingly, if we could . . .": Jeb Willenbring, e-mail to the author, 2 July 2005.

183   A few years ago Janet and Don Burleson: Dan Shaw, "Yes, That's Right, It's A Seeing-Eye *Horse*," *Newsweek* 11 November 2002, 20.

183 The Mind's Eye Foundation: 22 November 2007, <http://www. lisafittipaldi.com/foundation.htm>.

184 John Fago, who teaches people: Andrew Potok, *A Matter of Dignity: Changing the Lives of the Disabled* (New York: Bantam, 2002), 114.

184 Alex Truesdell makes chairs: Potok, 131–32.

184 "certainly not excluding . . .": Potok, 132.

184 "Blessed are they who talk . . .": "Blind Beatitudes," *Lilac Blind Foundation*, 5 June 2005, <http://lilacblindfoundation. org/news_information.php?id=66&flag=1>.

186 "I envy all who see things . . .": Kuusisto, 86.

186 "I remember walking home . . .": Coreen Faulkner, e-mail to the author.

187 "Perhaps humanity will manage . . .": Saramago, 229.

Chapter 9

191 "For more than thirty-five years . . .": Lusseyran, "Blindness: A New Revelation of the Light," 14 May 2005, <http://www. cygnusbooks.co.uk/features/blindness_jacques_lusseyran.htm.>.

191 "I truly feel that . . .": Lisa Fittipaldi.

191 "All the horror . . .": Griffin, 225.

191 blindness is the "wrapping": Hull, 205, 207.

191 "roses grow[ing] on the sheer banks . . .": Kuusisto, 179, 72–73.

192 Finally, in a hilarious account: Ryan Knighton, "Out of Sight," *Utne Magazine*, July–August 2005, 44.

192   "Fingertips seek out familiarity . . .": Harriet Welty Rochefort, "Paris Diary 6, November 2004—Eating in the Dark in Paris," 27 November 2007, <http://www.understandfrance.org/Diaries/ParisDiary6.htm>.

194   "a people's dream that died . . .": Nicholas Black Elk, *Black Elk Speaks* (as told through John G. Neihardt) (Lincoln: University of Nebraska Press, 1979) 1, 196–201.

194   "the darkness of men's eyes": Black Elk, xxi.

195   "the despotism of sight": Qtd in Sacks, 57.

196   "will not let life be": Olsen, *Yonnondio: From the Thirties* (New York: Delta/Seymour Lawrence, 1974), 37.

197   alcoholism "has been my most prolific teacher . . .": "The Spirituality of Addiction and Recovery," *Speaking of Faith* 27 July 2006, <speakingoffaith.publicradio.org/programs/recovery/index.shtml>.

198   "The cares of tomorrow . . .": W. Gordon Smith. "Come By the Hills," 5 August 2007, <http://www.mysongbook.de/msb/songs/c/comeby.html>.

Sources

Letters from Dennis Faulkner to Hattie Miller, 1936–38.

E-mails to the author from Mona Faulkner, Jeanne Adelmeyer, Elaine Willenbring, Coreen Faulkner, Jeb Willenbring, Chad McGuire, 2005–2007.

Interviews and conversations with Judy McGuire, Jeanne Adelmeyer, Elaine Willenbring, Dennis Faulkner, Coreen Faulkner, Mona Faulkner, Jeb Willenbring, Roys Willenbring. 2005–2007.

Adelmeyer, Jeanne. "My Father's Harmonica." Unpublished poem.

Akenson, Donald Harman. *The Irish Diaspora: A Primer*. Toronto: Meany, 1993.

Alexandria Citizen. 18 May 1905.

American Heritage Dictionary of the English Language 4th ed. New York: Houghton Mifflin, 2000.

Anderson, Tom, et al, eds. *Chronicle of America*. Mount Kisco, NY: Chronicle, 1989.

Barnhill, Susan. *Blind Student Earns M.D.* 2 April 2005. Station504.com. 14 May 2005 <http://www.station504.com/BlindMD.htm>.

Batson, Larry. *The Minneapolis Tribune*. 18 June 1981. 3B, 4B.

Betenbaugh, Helen, and Marjorie Procter-Smith. "Disabling the Lie: Prayers of Truth and Transformation." In Eisland and Saliers, *Human Disability and the Service of God: Reassessing Religious Practice*, 281–303.

SOURCES

Black Elk, Nicholas. *Black Elk Speaks.* (As told through John G. Neihardt.) Lincoln: University of Nebraska Press, 1979.

Blackhall, David Scott. *This House Had Windows.* New York: Obolensky, 1962.

Blassingame, John W., ed. *The Frederick Douglass Papers.* Series 1, vol. 1. New Haven: Yale University Press, 1979–1992.

"Blind Beatitudes." *Lilac Blind Foundation.* 5 June 2005 <http://lilacblind-foundation.org/ news_information.php?id=66&flag=1>.

"Blind Man Wows Faculty, Earns Medical Degree." *St. Cloud Times.* 3 April 2005. 9A.

Boland, Eavan. *An Origin like Water: Collected Poems 1967–1987.* New York: Norton, 1996.

———. "Famine Roads." In Hayden, *Irish Hunger,* 212–22.

Bolles, Richard Nelson. *What Color Is Your Parachute? A Practical Manual for Job-Hunters and Career Changes.* Berkeley: Ten-Speed, 1990, 2000.

Books Featuring Characters Who Are Visually Impaired. Iowa Braille School. 19 April 2005. <http://www.iowa-braille.k12.ia.us/bibliography_of_blind.html>.

Borges, Jorge Luis. "Blindness." In *The Art of the Personal Essay.* Ed. Phillip Lopate. New York: Anchor Books, 1994. 377–86.

Bradley, Eric. "Disability Is No Hindrance for Blind Teacher: Blindness Enhances Her Mission to Make Children Independent." *The Braille Monitor.* May 2003. <http://www.nfb.org/bm/bm03/bm0305/bm030505.htm>.

"Braille without Borders." *Climbing Blind Tibet Expedition.* 2004. Climbing Blind. 11 May 2005. <http://www.climbingblind.org/The%20Cause/braillewithoutborders.icm>.

Campbell, Stephen J. *The Great Irish Famine: Words and Images from the Famine Museum, Strokestown Park, County Roscommon.* Ireland: The Famine Museum, 1994.

Catlin, George. *Letter and Notes on the Manners, Customs, and Conditions of the North American Indians, Written during Eight Years' Travel*

SOURCES

(1832–39) amongst the Wildest Tribes of Indians in North America Vol. I and II. New York: Dover, 1973.

"Cause, The." *Climbing Blind Tibet Expedition.* 2004. Climbing Blind. 11 May 2005. <http://www.climbingblind.org/The%20Cause>.

Chapman, Robert L., ed. *Roget's International Thesaurus* 5th ed. New York: HarperCollins, 1992.

Christgau, John. *"Enemies": World War II Alien Internment.* Ames: Iowa State University Press, 1985.

Clark, Eleanor. *Eyes, Etc: A Memoir.* New York: Pantheon Books, 1977.

Coogan, Tim Pat. "The Lessons of the Famine for Today." In Hayden, *Irish Hunger*, 165–77.

Danielsen, Christopher. "More Perspectives on Blind Justice." Voice of the Nation's Blind. 6 May 2005. <http://www.voiceofthenationsblind. org/articles/131/more-perspectives-on-blind-justice>.

Davis, Graham. "The Historiography of the Irish Famine." In O'Sullivan, *Meaning of the Famine*, 15–39.

DelVecchio, Rick. "Blind Photographer's Vision Extends beyond Her Eyes." 18 February 2005. <http://www.nfbnet.org/pipermail/artbe-yondsightmuseums/2005/000102.html>.

Diner, Hasia R. *Erin's Daughters in America: Irish Immigrant Women in the Nineteenth Century.* Baltimore: Johns Hopkins University Press, 1983.

Donnelly, James S., Jr. *The Great Irish Potato Famine.* Gloucestershire: Sutton, 2001.

Donovan, Lauren. "Going Full Circle: Will the Return of Ancestral Lands Right an Old Wrong?" *The Bismarck Tribune.* Sunday, 22 May 2005. 1A, 7A.

DuBois, W. E. B. *The Souls of Black Folk.* Ed. David W. Blight and Robert Gooding-Williams. Boston: Bedford Books, 1997.

Eiesland, Nancy L. *The Disabled God: Toward a Liberatory Theology of Disability.* Nashville: Abingdon, 1994.

———. "Encountering the Disabled God." In *The Other Side.* (September/ October 2002): 10–15.

SOURCES

————, and Don E. Saliers, eds. *Human Disability and the Service of God: Reassessing Religious Practice*. Nashville: Abingdon, 1998.

Farrell, Bernadette. *Christ Be Our Light*. Portland: Oregon Catholic Press, 1994.

Fegan, Melissa. *Literature and the Irish Famine 1845–1919*. Oxford: Clarendon, 2002.

Fittipaldi, Lisa. *A Brush with Darkness: Learning to Paint after Losing My Sight*. 14 April 2005. <http://www.andrewwsmcmeel.com/products/?isbn=07040746936>.

Gallagher, Catherine, and Stephen Greenblatt. *Practicing New Historicism*. Chicago: University of Chicago Press, 2000.

Gallagher, Thomas. *Paddy's Lament: Ireland 1846–1847, Prelude to Hatred*. Orlando, FL: Harcourt Brace Jovanovich, 1982.

"Garrison Dam." *Mhanation.com*. 2004. Three Affiliated Tribes. 27 May 2005. <http://www.mhanation.com/main/history/history_garrison_dam.html>.

Germans from Russia: Children of the Steppe, Children of the Prairie, The. Prairie Public Broadcasting, 1999. Fargo, ND.

Gibbons, Luke. "Doing Justice to the Past." In Hayden, *Irish Hunger*, 258–70.

Gilman, Carolyn, and Mary Jane Schneider. *The Way to Independence*. St. Paul: Minnesota Historical Society Press, 1987.

Gold, Stephen. "Beyond Pity and Paternalism." *The Other Side*. (September/October 2002): 17–21.

Green, Dr. E. R. R. "The Great Famine (1845–1850)." In Moody and Martin, *Course of Irish History*. 263–74.

Greenfeld, Karl. "Blind to Failure." *Time*. 18 June 2001. 52.

Greer, Germaine. Interview by Joseph Kastner. *Women Writers Talking*. Ed. Janet Todd. New York: Holmes and Meier, 1983.

Griffin, John H. *Scattered Shadows: A Memoir of Blindness and Vision*. Maryknoll, NY: Orbis Books, 2004.

Grunwald, Henry. *Twilight: Losing Sight, Gaining Insight*. New York: Knopf, 1999.

SOURCES

Gwaltney, John L. *The Thrice Shy: Cultural Accommodation to Blindness and Other Disasters in a Mexican Community.* New York: Columbia University Press, 1970.

Hampl, Patricia. "Memory and Imagination." *I Could Tell You Stories.* New York: Norton, 1999. 21–37.

Hanson, Jeffrey R. "Introduction." In Wilson *Buffalo Bird Woman's Garden.* xi–xxiii.

Harle, Donald D. "The Dance Hall of the Santee Bottoms on the Fort Berthold Reservation, Garrison Reservoir, North Dakota." In Roberts, *River Basin Survey Papers,* 123–32.

Hayden, Tom. "The Famine of Feeling." In Hayden, *Irish Hunger,* 271–93.

———, ed. *The Irish Hunger: Personal Reflections on the Legacy of the Famine.* Boulder, CO: Roberts Rinehart, 1997.

———. *Irish on the Inside.* London: Verso, 2001.

Height, Joseph S. *Paradise on the Steppe: A Cultural History of the Kutschurgan, Beresan, and Liebental Colonists, 1804–1944.* Bismarck: North Dakota Historical Society of Germans from Russia, 1972.

Hine, Robert V. *Second Sight.* Berkeley: University of California Press, 1993.

Hull, John M. *Touching the Rock: An Experience of Blindness.* New York: Pantheon Books, 1990.

"Interview with Stephen Kuusisto, An." 30 May 2005. <http://www.randomhouse.com/boldtype/0398/kuusisto/interview.html>.

In the Mind of the Beholder. Director Karen Brown Davison. Produced by the Department of Communication, Stanford University. Videorecording, 1997.

Irish in America: The Long Journey Home. Directors Thomas Lennon and Mark Zwonitzer. Videocassette. Lennon Documentary Group, 1999.

Irish Pub Classics. Irish Records International. Vol. 3. Pembroke, MA. 2001.

Jernigan, Kenneth. "Blindness: Is History against Us?" 16 April 2005. <http://www. blind.net/bpbal1973.htm>.

SOURCES

"Joint Tribal Advisory Committee." *Mhanation.com*. 2004. Three Affiliated Tribes. 27 May 2005. <http://www.mhanation.com/main/history/history_jtac.html>.

Kennelly, Brendan. "My Dark Fathers." In Hayden, *Irish Hunger*, 245–47.

Kenny, Kevin. *The American Irish: A History*. New York: Pearson Education, 2000.

Killen, John, ed. *The Famine Decade: Contemporary Accounts 1841–1851*. Belfast: Blackstaff, 1995.

Kinealy, Christine. " 'The Famine Killed Everything': Living with the Memory of the Great Hunger." In Valone and Kinealy, *Ireland's Great Hunger*. 1–40.

———. "Potatoes, Providence, and Philanthropy: The Role of Private Charity during the Irish Famine." In O'Sullivan, *Meaning of the Famine*, 140–71.

Klein, Karl Matthias. *The History of Millerville, Douglas County, Minnesota, 1866–1930*. Millerville: Klein Company Store, 1930.

Knighton, Ryan. "Out of Sight." *Utne Magazine*, July/August 2005, 44.

Koestler, Frances A. *The Unseen Minority: A Social History of Blindness in the United States*. New York: McKay, 1976.

Kuusisto, Stephen. *Planet of the Blind*. New York: Dial, 1998.

Lawson, Michael L. *Dammed Indians: The Pick-Sloan Plan and the Missouri River Sioux, 1944–1980*. Norman: University of Oklahoma Press, 1982.

Leo, J. "Of Famine and Green Beer." *U.S. News and World Report*. 24 March 1997, 16.

"Letter That Started It All, The." *Climbing Blind Tibet Expedition*. 2004. 11 May 2005. <http://www.climbingblind.org/The%20Cause/the_letter.icm>.

Lloyd, David. "The Memory of Hunger." In Hayden, *Irish Hunger*, 32–47.

Lusseyran, Jacques. *And There Was Light: Autobiography of Jacques Lusseyran, Blind Hero of the French Resistance*. Trans. Elizabeth R. Cameron. New York: Parabola Books, 1998.

SOURCES

———. "Blindness: A New Revelation of the Light." 14 May 2005. <http://www.cygnusbooks.co.uk/features/blindnesss_jacques_lusseyran.htm>

"Mandan, The." *Mhanation.com*. 2004. Three Affiliated Tribes. 27 May 2005. <http://www.mhanation.com/main/history/history_mandan.html>.

McDonald, OSB, Sister M. Grace. *With Lamps Burning*. Saint Joseph, MN: Saint Benedict's Priory Press, 1957.

McFeely, William S. *Frederick Douglass*. New York: Norton, 1995.

"Melrose Man Braves Elements, Tests Limits at Iditarod." *St. Cloud Times*. 6 March 2005. 1B, 8B.

Metcalf, George. "Small Sites on and about Fort Berthold Indian Reservation, Garrison Reservoir, North Dakota." In Roberts, *River Basin Survey Papers*, 5–56.

———. "Star Village: A Fortified Historic Arikara Site in Mercer County, North Dakota." In Roberts, *River Basin Survey Papers*, 61–122.

Miller, Kerby, and Paul Wagner. *Out of Ireland: The Story of Irish Emigration to America*. Washington, DC: Elliot and Clark, 1994.

Mind's Eye Foundation, The. 22 November 2007. <http://www.lisafittipaldi.com/foundation.htm>.

Moloney, Mick. *Far from the Shamrock Shore: The Story of Irish–American Immigration through Song*. New York: Crown, 2002.

Moody, T. W., and F. X. Martin eds. *The Course of Irish History*. Dublin: Mercier, 1994. "A Chronology of Irish History." 425–81.

Morash, Christopher. "Making Memories: The Literature of the Irish Famine." In O'Sullivan, *Meaning of the Famine*, 40–55.

Morrison, Toni. *Song of Solomon*. New York: Penguin Books, 1977.

Murphy, Maureen, Maureen McCann Militta, Alan Singer. "Designing the New York State Great Irish Famine Curriculum Guide." In Valone and Kinealy, *Ireland's Great Hunger*. 361–92.

National Federation of the Blind. 7 March 2007. <http://www.nfb.org/nfb/Default.asp>.

Newell, J. Phillip. *Celtic Benediction: Morning and Night Prayer*. Grand Rapids, MI: Erdmans, 2000.

SOURCES

New Oxford Annotated Bible, The. New Revised Standard Edition. New York: Oxford University Press, 1994.

Nicholls, Horatio, and Edgar Leslie. "Among My Souvenirs." 25 October 2005. <http://www.reelclassics.com/Movies/BestYears/bestyears-souvenirs.htm>.

Nolan, Janet A. *Ourselves Alone: Women's Emigration from Ireland 1885–1920.* Lexington, Kentucky: University Press of Kentucky, 1989.

Nonpartisan League. Minnesota Historical Society. 10 March 2005. <http://www.mnhs.org/library/tips/history_topics/102nonpartisan.html>.

Ó Cathaoir, Brendan. *Famine Diary.* Dublin: Irish Academic, 1999.

O'Flaherty, Liam. *Famine: A Novel.* Boston: Godine, 1982.

Ó Gráda, Cormac. *The Great Irish Famine.* Cambridge: Cambridge University Press, 1995.

Oliver, Mary. "The Bright Eyes of Eleonora: Poe's Dream of Recapturing the Impossible." *Winter Hours: Prose, Prose Poems, and Poems.* Boston: Houghton Mifflin, 1999. 37–48.

Olsen, Tillie, "I Stand Here Ironing." *Tell Me a Riddle.* New York: Delta/Seymour Laurence, 1989. 1–12.

———. "Requa." *Iowa Review,* 1, no. 3 (Summer 1970): 54–74. Rpt. as "Requa-I" in *Best American Short Stories,* ed. Martha Foley and David Burnett, pp. 237–65. Boston: Houghton Mifflin, 1971.

———. *Silences.* New York: Feminist Press, 2003.

———. *Yonnondio: From the Thirties.* New York: Delta/Seymour Lawrence, 1974.

O'Reilly, Marie Whitla. "Works of Angels: Dublin Treasures Illuminate Life, Death and Resurrection." *National Catholic Reporter.* 15 April 2005. 4B, 5B.

O'Sullivan, Patrick, ed. *The Meaning of the Famine,* vol. 6. London: Leicester University Press, 1997.

Otis, D. S. *The Dawes Act and the Allotment of Indian Lands.* Ed. and intro. Francis Paul Prucha. Norman: University of Oklahoma Press, 1973.

Oxford English Dictionary. < http://www.oed.com/>.

SOURCES

Peck, Deborah. "Silent Hunger: The Psychological Impact of the Great Hunger." In Valone and Kinealy, *Ireland's Great Hunger*. 142–79.

Peters, Virginia. *Women of the Earth Lodge*. North Haven, CT: Anchor Books, 1995.

Pipher, Mary. *The Middle of Everywhere: The World's Refugees Come to Our Town*. New York: Harcourt, 2002.

Potok, Andrew. *A Matter of Dignity: Changing the World of the Disabled*. New York: Bantam Books. 2002.

Quinn, Peter. "In Search of the Banished Children: A Famine Journey." In Hayden, *Irish Hunger*, 143–56.

Regan, Ann. *Irish in Minnesota*. St. Paul: Minnesota Historical Society Press, 2002.

Reha, Bob. "North Dakota's First Capital Punishment Case in 100 Years Set to Begin in Fargo. <http://www.minnesota.publicradio.org/display/web/2006/05/13/nddeathpenalty>.

"Re: Turn a Blind Eye." *The Phrase Finder*. 22 February 2005. <http://www.phrases.org.uk/bulletin_board/8/messages/288.html>.

Rios, Delia M. "Indian Image Is Cast in a Chief's Portrait." *Star Tribune*. 24 November 2002. E5.

Roberts, Frank H. H., Jr., ed. *River Basin Survey Papers: Inter-Agency Archeological Salvage Program*. Vol. 6, no. 185. Washington, DC: U.S. Government Printing Office, 1963.

Rochefort, Harriet Welty. "Paris Diary 6, November 2004—Eating in the Dark in Paris." 27 November 2007. <http://www.understandfrance.org/Diaries/ParisDiary6.htm>.

Sachs, Jeff. "The End of Poverty." *Time*. 11 March 2005, 42–54.

Sacks, Oliver. *An Anthropologist on Mars: Seven Paradoxical Tales*. New York: Knopf, 1995.

———. "A Neurologist's Notebook: The Mind's Eye." *The New Yorker*. 28 July 2003, 48–59.

Said, Edward W. *Orientalism*. New York: Pantheon. 1978.

Saint-Exupéry, Antoine de. *The Little Prince*. Trans. Katherine Woods. New York: Harcourt Brace Jovanovich, 1982.

SOURCES

Saramago, Jose. *Blindness*. Trans. Giovanni Pontiero. New York: Harcourt Brace, 1998.

Satchell, Michael. "Trashing the Reservations?" *U.S. News & World Report.* 114, no. 1 (January 1993). 6 July 2005. <http://www.nathannewman. org/EDIN/.race/.racefile/.jan-feb/envi-race1/nativeAm.html>.

Schroeder, Frederic K. "Orientation and Mobility, Competence and Hypocrisy." 25 July 2006. <http://www.nfb.org/bm/bm03/bm0309/ Bm030908.htm>.

Sexton, Sean, and Christine Kenealy. *The Irish: A Photohistory*. New York: Thomas and Hudson, 2002.

Shaw, Dan. "Yes, That's Right, It's a Seeing-Eye *Horse*." *Newsweek*. 11 November 2002, 20.

Shields, Chris. "Utah Reservation Might Store Nuclear Waste." *St. Cloud Times*. 10 September 2005, 3A.

Smith, G. Hubert. *Like-a-Fishhook Village and Fort Berthold Garrison Reservoir North Dakota*. Washington: National Park Service, U.S. Dept. of the Interior, 1972.

Smith, W. Gordon. "Come by the Hills." 5 August 2007. <http://www. mysongbook.de/msb/songs/c/comeby.html>.

"Snow Country Prison: Interned in North Dakota." *North Dakota Museum of Art*. 1998. 5 February 2005. <http://www.ndmoa.com/template. cfm?page=SnowCountryPrison>.

"Spirituality of Addiction and Recovery, The." *Speaking of Faith*. 27 July 2006. <speakingoffaith.publicradio.org/programs/recovery/index. shtml>.

Springfield, Tom. "A World of Our Own." Columbia DB 7532.

"Stephen Kuusisto." *The Ohio State University*. 3 June 2005. <http://people. cohums.ohio-state.edu/kuusisto1>.

tenBroek, Jacobus, and Floyd W. Matson. *Hope Deferred: Public Welfare and the Blind*. Berkeley: University of California Press, 1959.

"Touch the Universe: Creating Cosmic Images for the Blind to 'See'." *St. Cloud Visitor*. 11 September 2003.

Tweton, D. Jerome. "The Fort Lincoln Internment Camp." *North Dakota Humanities Council*. 5 February 2005. <http://www.nd-humanities. org/html/wwiiinternment.html>.

SOURCES

United States Federal Census, 1880, 1900, 1920. 16 April 2005. <http://www.ancestrylibrary.com/default.aspx>.

Valone, David A., and Christine Kinealy. *Ireland's Great Hunger: Silence, Memory, and Commemoration.* Lanham: University Press of America, 2002.

VanDevelder, Paul. *Coyote Warrior: One Man, Three Tribes, and the Trial That Forged a Nation.* New York: Little, Brown. 2004.

Viola, Herman J. *Little Bighorn Remembered: The Untold Story of Custer's Last Stand.* New York: Times Books, 1999.

Wagner, Sally. *How Do You Kiss a Blind Girl?* Springfield, IL: Thomas, 1986.

"Wahanee: An Indian Girl's Story Told by Herself to Gilbert L. Wilson." In *North Dakota History: Journal of the Northern Plains*, 38, nos. 1 and 2 (Winter/Spring 1971). Rpt. in Peter Nabokov, ed. *Native American Testimony.* New York: Viking, 1991.

Wall, Maureen. "The Age of the Penal Laws (1691–1778)." In Moody and Martin, *Course of Irish History.* 217–31.

Wells, H. G. "The Country of the Blind." *The Complete Short Stories of H.G. Wells.* New York: St. Martin's, 1971. 167–92.

Weihenmayer, Erik. *Touch the Top of the World: A Blind Man's Journey to Climb Farther Than the Eye Can See.* New York: Dutton, 2001.

When Ireland Starved. Director Joseph Dunn. Performer Peter Kelly. Videocassette. Films for the Humanities, 1993.

Wilson, Gilbert A. *Buffalo Bird Woman's Garden: Agriculture of the Hidatsa Indians.* St. Paul: Minnesota Historical Society Press, 1987.

Wolfe, Kathi. "Fighting Stereotypes: 'Supercrips' Images Pose Unrealistic Expectations on Disabled People." *Minneapolis Star Tribune.* 6 July 2001. 19A.

Woodham-Smith, Cecil. *The Great Hunger: Ireland 1845–1849.* New York: Harper and Row, 1962.

Yeates, Ray. "My Famine." In Hayden, *Irish Hunger*, 191–202.

Zinsser, William, ed. "Introduction." In *Inventing the Truth: The Art and Craft of Memoir.* Boston: Houghton Mifflin, 1998. 1–22.